DATE DUE

FE__			
__			
NO - 6 08			

DEMCO 38-296

MIC
FBA   st
and

He
grad
prof
Acup
retir

He
subj

ACUPUNCTURE

An introductory guide to the technique and its benefits

Michael Nightingale

Illustrated by
Shaun Williams

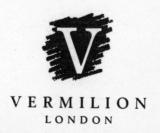

VERMILION
LONDON

:Donald Optima
)1
Optima
Reprinted 1994

1 3 5 7 9 10 8 6 4 2

This edition published in the United Kingdom in 1997 by
Vermilion, an imprint of Ebury Press

Random House UK Ltd
Random House
20 Vauxhall Bridge Road
London SW1V 2SA

Random House Australia (Pty) Ltd
20 Alfred Street, Milsons Point, Sydney
New South Wales 2016, Australia

Random House New Zealand Limited
18 Poland Rd, Glenfield,
Aukland 10, New Zealand

Random House, South Africa (Pty) Limited
Endulini, 5A Jubilee Road, Parktown 2193,
South Africa

Random House UK Limited Reg. No. 954009

A CIP catalogue record for this book is available from the
British Library.

ISBN 0 09 181518 5

Printed and bound in Great Britain by Mackays of Chatham

Papers used by Vermilion are natural, recyclable products
made from wood grown in sustainable forests.

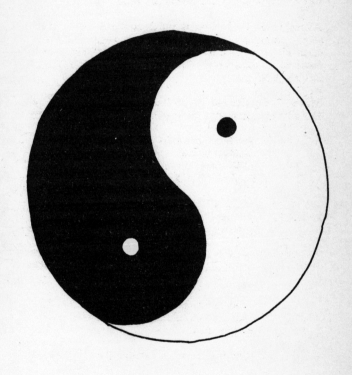

CONTENTS

1. THINKING ABOUT ACUPUNCTURE

'There are more things in heaven and earth, Horatio, than are dreamt of in your philosophy' (Hamlet, Act 1. Sc V)

WHAT IS ACUPUNCTURE?

Acupuncture consists of inserting very fine needles into the skin at certain specified points, selected in accordance with the patient's disease and basic constitution. The needles are normally made from stainless steel.

The points at which the needles are inserted are called acupuncture points, acupoints or acupores. They are very precisely located, and have to be carefully chosen by considering a number of factors, many of which will be explained further on in this book.

Acupuncture is part of a complete system of medicine which has been practised in China for many thousands of years. This medicine included acupuncture, herbal medicine, manipulative therapy, diet, relaxation and special exercises. Acupuncture was used mostly for the treatment of superficial diseases such as skin problems, ulcers, wounds, headaches, coughs, disorders involving phlegm and digestive upsets, as well as some mental illnesses.

Occasionally conditions which we now regard as infectious were also treated with acupuncture. Diseases involving the vital organs, however, were more often treated with herbs, and musculoskeletal complaints were mainly treated with massage and manipulation.

Today, acupuncture is widely used and there have been many recent developments in the field. Sometimes it is used in conjunction with manipulative techniques or with homoeopathy, as it combines with them well.

THE NEEDLES

Acupuncture needles were not always made of stainless steel, of course. In the early practice of acupuncture, thorns, bamboo splints and pieces of sharpened stone were used. Iron needles were manufactured during the Iron Age, and later needles were made from the precious metals of gold and silver. These were thought to be superior, and were usually reserved for the aristocracy. Some practitioners believed that gold and silver needles had special qualities: gold was thought to stimulate, while silver was said to have a sedating action. A few acupuncturists still believe this even today but most now use only stainless steel needles — which, of course, are considerably cheaper! However, needles made of gold, silver, copper and zinc are all used in particular cases because they are thought to possess especial qualities of stimulation or sedation.

The word 'acupuncture' itself is comparatively new, and is probably derived from the latin *acus* (a needle) and *punctum* (the past participle of the verb *pungere*, meaning to puncture or pierce).

However, it is not always necessary to use needles in

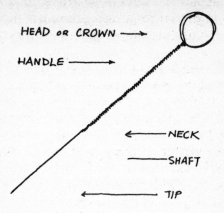

HEAD or CROWN ⟶

HANDLE ⟶

⟵ NECK

⟶ SHAFT

⟵ TIP

order to treat 'acupuncture' points. Traditionally, pressure or massage with a finger, and heat from a burning herb, were also employed as methods of stimulating or activating the points. In modern times, electricity, sound, ultrasound, microwave, magnetism and laser have all been used with varying degrees of success.

Although acupuncture without needles is something of a contradiction in terms, the words 'acupressure', 'laserpuncture' and 'sonopuncture' are frequently used, and conveniently refer to the treatment of acupuncture points by finger pressure, laser or sound.

WHERE DID ACUPUNCTURE COME FROM?

It is generally thought that acupuncture began in China, although it was also certainly practised in other oriental countries in very early times. Documents over 1,000 years old have been found in Sri Lanka, depicting the acupuncture points of the elephant.

Early stone and quartz 'needles' or probes which were used in the treatment of ailments have been unearthed in

China. This treatment was termed 'bian', and was the precursor of acupuncture; it was practised more than a thousand years BC. Bone and bamboo needles were also used, and excavations from the ruins of the Yin Dynasty (which existed more than 3,000 years ago) have confirmed that acupuncture was being practised at least as long ago as that. From about 400 BC onwards, metal needles began to be used.

HOW DID ACUPUNCTURE START?

Nobody knows for certain how acupuncture started. It is most likely that it evolved as a result of careful observation, experimentation and deduction. The ancient Chinese physicians may have noticed that some illnesses or disorders resulted in certain points or specific areas on the skin becoming spontaneously sensitive. They may also have discovered that massaging or pressing on these points brought relief from symptoms. At first this pressure would probably have been applied with the fingers or hand, or some other part of the body; later, stones would have been used, and later still needles.

Since acupuncture is so ancient, it is not surprising that there are many legends surrounding it. One legend tells how soldiers, wounded by arrows, were cured from diseases they had suffered from for years. We can imagine a soldier going to war, and many years later returning to his doctor. The doctor asks, 'Have you come for treatment?' 'Oh no', replies the soldier. 'Since I was shot by an arrow, my backache has completely disappeared!'

Another legend claims extraterrestrial sources for the origin of acupuncture. It is said, for example, that the legendary Emperor Fu Hsi, one of the founders of the art of healing, had all wisdom bestowed upon him by superior beings. Some modern scientists have speculated that the Earth may even have been visited by voyagers from distant planets who brought with them, among other things, the knowledge of acupuncture.

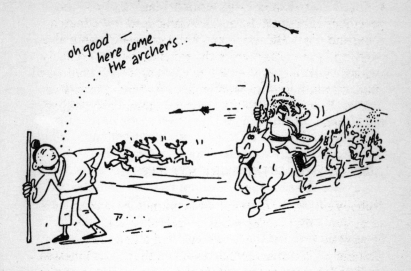

WHEN DID ACUPUNCTURE COME TO THE WEST?

It may seem surprising, but acupuncture began its spread all over the world some 3,000 years ago. In the eleventh century AD, the famous Persian physician Avicenna was writing about 'energic channels', or meridians.

Primitive forms of acupuncture are still practised in many countries. Eskimos still use sharpened stones to treat illnesses, and some Arab physicians will cauterize particular points, especially on the ear. The Bantus scratch certain areas on the skin to allay illness, and there is a tribe in Brazil which uses small darts shot from blowpipes to treat disease. Writings from Egypt dating back over 3,000 years describe a system of energy channels similar to the Chinese acupuncture system.

The first person to describe acupuncture in the West was probably Willem Ten Rhyne, a Dutch physician living in the sixteenth century. The first edition of the medical journal *The Lancet* in 1823 carried an article on the subject, and numerous nineteenth-century doctors and scientists investigated it. Nevertheless, acupuncture remained virtually unknown in the West until the present century.

Ironically, it was at a time when acupuncture was being suppressed in China following the advent of western medicine, in 1939, that a French diplomat, Georges Soulie de Morant, who had made a detailed study of the subject in China, published a French acupuncture manual. This gave acupuncture a tremendous boost in France. Unfortunately, however, de Morant died a disillusioned man after the same people whom he had taught turned on him and invoked the law to prevent him from practising.

In most western countries, the established medical profession resisted the advance of acupuncture. The moment of change came in 1972, when President Nixon visited the People's Republic of China, and the journalist James Reston described how his post-operative pain was eased by acupuncture when conventional drugs had failed. The subsequent observation of major surgery being carried out under acupuncture analgesia confronted the medical profession with incontrovertible evidence of its efficacy.

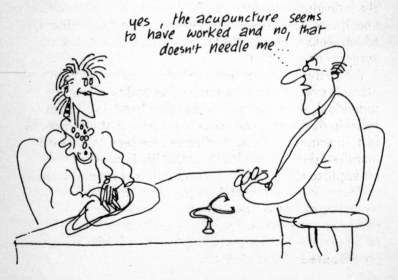

Since then a slow but rather grudging acceptance of acupuncture has begun to evolve. However, there are still large numbers of doctors who regard it merely as a limited method of pain control, and many who know nothing about the subject at all.

At the time of writing there are major acupuncture associations in most European countries and the Americas. Acupuncture is also widely practised in the USSR, and is becoming increasingly popular in the Arab world. A vigorous acupuncture association has been set up in Pakistan, and in India it is now well established. In Sri Lanka it is particularly popular, and the island has become world-famous as a centre of acupuncture thanks to the untiring efforts of one of its greatest exponents, Professor Jayasuriya.

HOW DOES ACUPUNCTURE DIFFER FROM ORDINARY MEDICINE?

The difference between acupuncture and conventional or 'allopathic' medicine is vast indeed. The very basis of acupuncture, which is primarily concerned with regulating the individual's life force, body energy or ch'i (pronounced chee), is quite different from that of allopathic medicine, which seeks to change the body by chemical substances, surgery or radioactivity.

Allopathic medicine tends to have a somewhat negative attitude towards the inherent healing ability of the individual. Acupuncture, on the other hand, has a firm belief in this power, and seeks to enhance it at all times. In fact, in acupuncture, acute diseases are seen as outward manifestations of the vitality of this life force as it attempts to rid the body of harmful influences and toxins.

Energy is vibration, and acupuncture works by correcting disharmonious vibration. Conventional medicine, on the other hand, imposes its own disease picture on the body in an attempt to force it into a preconceived notion of health.

Even the concepts of health are different: acupuncture sees health as a complete mental, emotional, social and physical well-being; whereas allopathy sees it as the mere absence of clinical symptoms. In acupuncture, emotional ill-health is regarded as the prime cause of disease; in conventional medicine it is ignored, or masked with tranquillizers or mind-altering drugs.

The acupuncture practitioner sees the patient as an individual, and the symptoms only as a signpost to treatment. The conventional physician, on the other hand, sees the symptoms as the most important factor and may even completely ignore the patient's individuality.

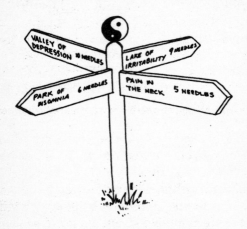

According to the philosophy behind acupuncture, disease is the result of a failure to conform to the laws of nature, either by the individual or by society. It therefore seeks to educate people so that they can see how and why they became ill in the first place. This contrasts with conventional medicine, which sees the cause of illness of something outside the individual and therefore beyond his or her control.

There are, of course, exceptions to some of these statements, but on the whole they represent an accurate description of the differences between acupuncture and conventional medicine.

ACUPUNCTURE	CONVENTIONAL MEDICINE
Patient orientated	Disease orientated
Non-invasive	Often invasive
Has no ill-effects	Has ill-effects
Very safe	Often unsafe
Vitalistic	Mechanistic
Energic	Physico-chemical
Disease a learning process	Disease an enemy
Disease the result of wrong habits	Disease an enemy which attacks
Cure is slow and deep	Cure often rapid and superficial
Holistic	Symptom specific
Promotes positive health	Health is absence of disease
Egalitarian: promotes self-responsibility	Authoritarian: requires surrender of patient

Comparison of acupuncture with western medicine

TAO, AND YIN AND YANG

Chinese medicine is often difficult for westerners to understand because its philosophy is completely different from that of western medicine, and its terminology reflects a different concept of physiology, health and disease.

The Tao is the 'Way' which maintains and orders the entire universe. It pervades all things, yet is unknowable. Creation was brought about by the expression by the Tao of the two complementary forces 'yin' and 'yang'. Yin and yang may be understood as interior and exterior, dark and light, or any other pair of complementary qualities. A fuller list of yin/yang correspondences is given in the table on page 20.

It is the right balance of yin and yang that is responsible for the harmonious functioning of the universe, including mankind. Humans stand between heaven and earth. According to Lao Tzu, the greatest classical exponent of

YIN	YANG
Cold	Hot
Earth	Heaven
Moon	Sun
Damp	Dry
Dark	Light
Passive	Active
Feminine	Masculine
Deep/interior	Superficial/exterior
Solid organs	Hollow organs
Front	Back

Some yin/yang correspondences

Tao, 'Man follows the laws of earth, earth follows the laws of heaven, heaven follows the laws of Tao, and Tao follows the laws of its intrinsic nature.'

People, however, do not always conform to this natural order of things, and therein is spelt disharmony and disease. Like everything else, the body energy or ch'i must reflect the correct and harmonious balance of yin and yang. It is the imbalance of yin and yang within the body which is synonymous with disease.

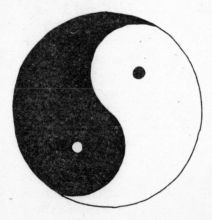

HEALTH - BALANCE OF YIN AND YANG

The Chinese were particularly concerned with the weather and climatic factors since these could, at times, be very harsh. They realized that the harmonious balance of yin and yang could be upset by prolonged exposure to extreme climatic conditions. More insidious still, they believed, was the harmful effect of damaging emotions such as anger, fear, jealousy, worry or grief.

The Chinese were also (and still are) very interested in food, and saw clearly the connection between diet and health. They analyzed their food, not in terms of chemical composition as we do in the West today, but in terms of yin and yang: the food's heating or cooling effect, and stimulating or sedating action.

The Chinese were aware of other factors, but these were always seen in the light of their cosmological beliefs and understanding. Today, we are once again beginning to learn what the Chinese realized many thousands of years ago: that disease is mostly the result of wrong living, and our failure to concern ourselves with the promotion of health. To a large extent we choose and create our own illnesses. The old way of thinking has caused us to be hell-bent on curing disease; the 'acupuncture' way is to live harmoniously so that disease is prevented in the first place.

2.
COULD ACUPUNCTURE HELP ME?

WHO SHOULD HAVE ACUPUNCTURE?

Some diseases respond particularly well to acupuncture, and these are mostly the ones which we describe as 'functional' — in other words, ones where structural or organic change has not taken place.

Obviously, diseases which do not respond well to conventional medicine, such as migraine, frozen shoulder, headache, impotence, asthma, many kinds of skin problems and muscular aches and pains are the most suitable for acupuncture treatment. Life-threatening conditions such as acute appendicitis or meningitis are the least suitable, although in the People's Republic of China many cases of appendicitis have been satisfactorily treated with acupuncture. Some conditions for which acupuncture is considered particularly suitable are listed overleaf.

Pain, whether acute or chronic, often responds dramatically to acupuncture. This is why it is important

asthma	arthritis	constipation
diarrhoea	indigestion	high blood pressure
low blood pressure	lack of energy	migraine
headaches	impotence	failure to conceive
menstrual disorders	neuralgia	depression
joint pains	back pains	sinusitis
phobias	sciatica	poor appetite
skin problems	haemorrhoids	insomnia
water retention	tinnitus	

Some conditions for which acupuncture is recommended

that the practitioner is properly qualified and is able to distinguish between painful conditions where acupuncture is advisable, and those where some other treatment should be provided as well.

ACUPUNCTURE: YOUR QUESTIONS ANSWERED

Do I need to be ill to have acupuncture?

No! Traditionally the Chinese doctor and his patients were much more concerned with prevention than cure. In fact, for some period of time, the Chinese doctor was only paid by his patients while they were well. If anyone became ill it was considered to be the doctor's fault, and the patient had to be restored to health without payment.

We have become accustomed to six-monthly dental checks, yet never consider the importance of having a complete body check. An annual check by an acupuncturist is a good investment, and goes a long way towards preventing problems in the future.

Are there people who should not have acupuncture?

Yes, there are some people who should not have acupuncture. Needles are not normally used on babies and

young children, though a skilful acupuncturist can make
the treatment acceptable. A better method of treating
acupuncture points in these cases is with laser or massage.

Extremely weak and very old people and those who are
unduly nervous as well as those who are particularly
frightened of needles are better treated by some other
method, such as laser.

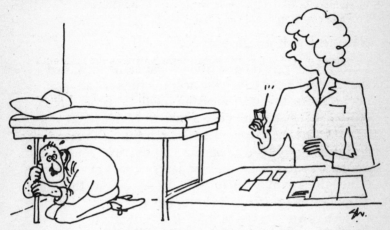

*Those who are particularly frightened of needles are better
treated by some other method...*

There are some conditions which do not respond as well
to acupuncture. They include cancer, severe infections,
heart disease, muscular dystrophy, venereal disease,
motor neurone disease, and any cases where surgery is
clearly indicated, such as appendicitis. For most of these
diseases, acupuncture may be usefully employed as a
supplement to other forms of treatment.

It must not be forgotten that acupuncture does not
really treat named diseases as such, but instead enhances
the general health and well-being of the individual. That's
why, although acupuncture is certainly not a 'cure-all',
there are really no conditions where it is not of some value.

Are there times when I should not have acupuncture?

It is better to defer acupuncture if you are so busy that you cannot afford the time to relax after the treatment. It is not ideal to have acupuncture during menstruation, if you are taking steroids, or have just started a course of drug therapy.

Should I ask my doctor?

Ideally, your general practitioner should be consulted so that he or she can notify the acupuncturist of any important facts concerning your medical history which otherwise they might not be aware of. Moreover, if you normally attend a doctor, it seems courteous to mention that you are thinking of having acupuncture. Many GPs are only too happy for their patients to have acupuncture if they think it might help, provided, of course, that the acupuncture practitioner is properly qualified.

Doctors are allowed to refer their patients to non-medical acupuncturists. Unfortunately, however, some prefer to send patients to medical colleagues who have done a short course in acupuncture, even though these may not be adequately trained. And some GPs regrettably know nothing at all about acupuncture, and so cannot sensibly advise their patients about it.

As you can see, it's something of a Catch 22! If your doctor is unfavourably disposed towards acupuncture, he or she won't refer you and might be annoyed that you suggested it. Even if they are favourably disposed, they might not send you to the best person. As things stand at present, it is recognized practice for patients to consult an acupuncturist independently of their GP, but to inform them if possible or if the acupuncturist advises it.

Some GPs actually suggest acupuncture to patients, and in these cases a good relationship between the doctor and acupuncturist can be established.

Why do some doctors not approve of acupuncture?

It is sometimes difficult for professional people, who have studied for many years and subsequently lived with a particular system, to adjust to new ideas. Nevertheless, more and more doctors are becoming interested in acupuncture, and in other forms of medicine which are different from that in which they qualified.

Some doctors do not like other practitioners treating their patients because it makes them feel threatened or undermined. They may have a genuine sense of responsibility for their patients which they think is not being properly discharged if an unknown person is treating them. Improved communication will eventually solve this, though it will undoubtedly take time.

Finding a practioner

Names and addresses of qualified acupuncturists can be obtained from official acupuncture associations such as the British Acupuncture Association or the British Acupuncture Council (see pages 105 - 109)

What do I need to do before seeing an acupuncturist?

Very little! As already discussed, try to avoid making an appointment when you are very busy. Don't have a very strenuous exercise programme just before the visit, and do not have a heavy meal or very hot bath beforehand. Wear suitable underclothing so that you can remove your outer garments without embarrassment.

The table overleaf indicates some items you should avoid wearing when going for acupuncture treatment.

DON'T WEAR
<ul><li>Perfume</li><li>Tight clothing</li><li>Heavy make-up</li><li>Jewellery</li><li>Watch</li><li>Deodorant</li></ul>

What not to wear during treatment

Does this mean I shall have to undress?

It is unlikely that acupuncturists would normally be prepared to treat patients who are fully dressed. This is because they need to examine and feel various parts of the body. Exceptions to this are sometimes made in the case of people who have acupuncture to help them give up smoking.

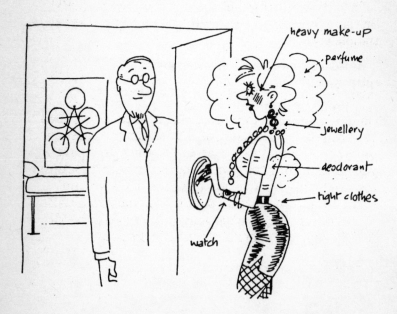

I don't like needles!

There are very few people who actually *enjoy* having needles put into them, but acupuncture is almost painless, and the small amount of discomfort is well worthwhile in most cases.

However, if you have a serious hang-up about needles, most acupuncturists are more than willing to use one or other of the alternatives already mentioned (page 25). Other methods to treat acupuncture points include massage, laser, microwave, electrical stimulation, sound, ultrasound, magnetism, light, heat and touch (see Chapter 8, pages 89-94).

Can acupuncture be dangerous?

Crossing the road is not without danger so we cannot in all honesty say that there is no danger in acupuncture. However, there is no inherent danger such as there is with drugs or surgery.

Provided the treatment is carried out by a properly qualified practitioner, acupuncture can be regarded as completely safe.

Are the needles properly sterilized?

As long as you go to a recognized practitioner, such as those on the Register of British Acupuncturists under the British Acupuncture Council (see page 27), you have nothing to worry about. All such practitioners are bound by a very strict code of ethics, and apart from the question of sterility, you can also be assured that their professional conduct will be all that is expected from a medical practitioner.

What about AIDS?

The virus associated with AIDS is relatively easily
destroyed, and all proper sterilization procedures are more
than adequate to ensure that there is absolutely no
possibility of transmitting AIDS. (Acupuncture has indeed
been used in several countries for the treatment of AIDS,
and has proved to be effective.)

Are there any side-effects?

There are no inherent side-effects. A few minor problems
may occur, but most of them are very rare. Minor bruising
is one of the most common, and may cause a slight
swelling and discolouration. This normally disappears
after a few days; and if arnica ointment (available from
most chemists) is applied at the time, any slight
discomfort is minimized.

A broken needle is an acupuncturist's nightmare, but it
is such a rare occurrence that it can be disregarded. By
regularly replacing needles and by not inserting them up
to the hilt, practitioners avoid this problem.

Things to avoid before having acupuncture

Do not wear heavy make-up or any scent. Deodorants,
talcum powder, after-shave and other cosmetics should
also be avoided since these will prevent the acupuncturist
from making an accurate diagnosis. They may also
aggravate the condition of another patient who happens to
be allergic to them.

Do not take any drugs unless it is absolutely necessary,
and in that case make sure that the acupuncturist knows.
A hot bath, strenuous exercise and sexual intercourse
should also be avoided just prior to acupuncture.

Do not squeeze your appointment between other
engagements as this will prevent you from getting the best
out of the treatment.

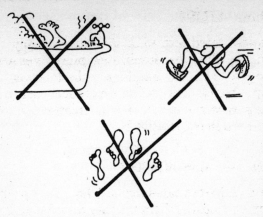

Avoid certain activities prior to acupuncture

What will the acupuncturist want to know?

Usually, the acupuncturist will want to know all your past medical history, and will be particularly interested in the season of the year when past problems occurred, the time of day when you felt better or worse, and when you finally recovered. Similar questions will be asked about your present problem, as well as how you are affected by heat, cold, dryness, damp and the wind.

The acupuncturist will certainly be interested in your emotional state, too, and will want to know about your relationships with parents, children, spouse, friends, employer, fellow workers and so on.

Other things you may be asked about include your family's medical history, the results of any relevant tests you might have had, your diet, including food likes and dislikes, your general lifestyle, and what sort of recreation and exercise you take.

How long will the treatment last?

On your first visit, if a treatment is included as well as a consultation and examination, the whole session will probably last about one hour. Subsequent visits are shorter, usually 30-45 minutes.

Sometimes the acupuncture treatment itself only lasts for 10 or 15 minutes. However, you will probably be in the surgery for at least half an hour, as the acupuncturist will need to ask you a few questions and examine you at each visit.

What will actually happen?

Many people are put off going for acupuncture because they simply have no idea what is likely to happen. We are always unnerved by the unknown. (In fact the unknown is far worse than the dreaded needles!) Be assured that acupuncturists are fully professional people whose aim is to help you as much as they can with the minimum of discomfort.

The acupuncturist will examine you, and this will include observing how you walk, stand, sit and talk. Your face will be looked at very closely to note your complexion, and to try and detect any odours or observe anything about you that might lead to a diagnosis. The tongue is especially important, so do not feel embarrassed at holding it out. Various points on the body may be gently touched to see if they are sensitive, as may your abdomen. In all probability your blood pressure will be taken, and the acupuncturist is also likely to examine your eyes.

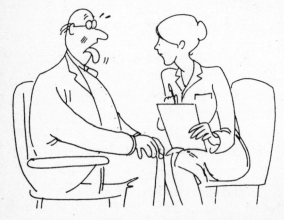

Do not feel embarrassed at holding out your tongue

When all this has been completed and you are in a comfortable position, a few acupuncture needles will be carefully inserted into the chosen points. The arms and legs, including the hands and feet, are the favourite places for the needles, but there are very few parts of the body which are 'no-go' areas. The genital area, however, is seldom used; other points which are never needled include the navel and the nipples.

How many treatments will I need?

This will depend on a host of different factors, including your inherent vitality and powers of recovery, how long you have had the problem, how serious it is, and what other problems you have.

Generally speaking between three and six treatment sessions clear up most conditions, but long-standing complaints may take considerably longer.

Will the treatments be painful?

None of us likes pain, and it is always a source of anxiety to prospective patients that the acupuncture treatment might be painful. In fact, acupuncture is almost painless — when the needle is inserted you usually feel just a tiny sting like the bite of an ant. Manipulation of the needle by the acupuncturist is occasionally a little painful if a nerve is being irritated.

Acupuncture needles are very fine and are inserted with great skill. The experience cannot be compared with the familiar injections you might have received from your doctor or in a hospital. Those injections are carried out with much thicker needles, the site of injection is not accurately defined, and the material injected often causes pain.

How much will it cost?

Obviously, this will depend upon how many treatments you require as well as where and by whom you are being treated. In larger cities, for example, fees are about 30 per cent higher than they are in the provinces. At the time of going to print, the current rates for treatment range from £15 to £30 per session. Usually, there is a consultation fee, but most practitioners charge this only on the first visit. A consultation fee is normally similar to a treatment fee.

Most practitioners are prepared to make an adjustment for those who cannot afford to pay the full fee, but in general fees are kept low so that ordinary people can afford treatment. Compared with standard medical fees, acupuncture fees are usually very modest.

In London and a few other places, there are college clinics which offer treatment at a reduced fee. The British College of Acupuncture (page 105) does this. All patients are supervised by a fully qualified acupuncturist. The students who carry out the treatment are already qualified in some branch of medicine and will have spent more than a year studying acupunture.

Will the cure be permanent?

It would be dishonest to say that all cures are permanent. However, in most cases, where a cure is possible, it will be permanent or at least very long-lasting.

Problems can recur if treatment is abandoned prematurely, or if the patient continues to indulge in bad habits which may have brought on the problem in the first place. For example, if you smoke tobacco and suffer from lung problems or circulatory disease, these are almost certain to return if you continue to smoke.
Acupuncture may work miracles at times, but it cannot do the impossible!

Acupuncturists distrust the word 'cure', because their kind of medicine works by enhancing the general vitality, so that patients are in fact cured by their own healing powers.

Is the treatment here as good as in China?

It would be inappropriate to say that treatment was either better or worse in China than in the West. Treatments vary from practitioner to practitioner, and generally treatment in the UK is as good as the best available in China.

Are gold and silver needles better than stainless steel ones?

There has been considerable discussion about this matter and no firm conclusions have been reached. Most acupuncturists regard stainless steel needles as being quite as good as gold or silver needles. If you particularly wish to have needles made from 'nobler' metals this is usually possible, but you might have to pay for them!

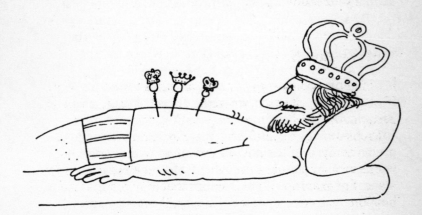

How many needles will I need?

This will depend on the practitioner's diagnosis and judgment about how to treat you. Usually about eight needles are used, but the number can vary from one to about twenty.

Do the needles contain anything?

Acupuncture needles are solid, and they do not contain any medication.

The only exception to this is in homoeopuncture (see page 93) which is not widely practised. In homoeopuncture the needle is dipped into the relevant homoeopathic remedy before insertion.

Do acupuncturists give any other kind of treatment?

Yes. All acupuncturists use moxa which is a method of applying heat to acupuncture points. Nearly all acupuncturists use electrical stimulation, and some use magnets, laser, sound, ultrasound, colour, pressure or even microwave to treat the acupuncture points. One of the newer techniques is that of pulsors, in which the special energy created by a crystal is used to activate the acupuncture point.

In addition, all members of the British Acupuncture Association, for example, are qualified in some other branch of medicine, and where appropriate will make use of such skills or refer you to a doctor who can undertake the treatment you require. For example, osteopathic treatment might be given in conjunction with the acupuncture if there was a musculoskeletal disorder.

Will the treatment be the same each time?

This is most unlikely, for the simple reason that you can change from treatment to treatment. However, the treatments will probably be very similar. In a few instances the identical treatment will be repeated, and sometimes an entirely different treatment might be tried.

How do I find the best practitioner for me?

Provided you select a properly qualified and registered practitioner you will have an acupuncturist whose professional ability is beyond question.

Of course, in every profession, one finds lazy, inefficient and discourteous people. Fortunately, these are very rare. And don't forget that, unlike most other medical practitioners, acupuncturists are paid direct by the patient. This means that unless they are efficient, courteous and understanding, they are unlikely to prosper.

Sometimes it just happens that two people do not get along well together. This is not an adverse reflection on either the doctor or the patient, but if this happens you should change to another practitioner. Acupuncturists, however, are trained to understand people, and are usually sympathetic or empathetic to the patient for whom they are anxious to do their best.

Should I feel the benefit immediately?

Sometimes this happens, particularly where pain is the predominant feature of the complaint. In many cases, however, the benefit is not really experienced for a few days and may not be noticed until after a second or third treatment.

In a few chronic cases it is necessary to have a long series of treatments before any benefit is felt.

How will I feel after the treatment?

Immediately after the treatment you might feel very relaxed and lightheaded. This is a good sign that the acupuncture has been effective. Some people feel very tired for a day or two after treatment, but the onset of this tiredness is often on the day after the treatment itself. Again, this is a good sign.

As far as your symptoms are concerned, on very rare occasions they may actually be worse after the first treatment. This is also usually a good sign, and you should arrange to have a second treatment as soon as possible. This second treatment will probably return you to your original state, and after subsequent sessions you will start to recover.

What should I do if I feel ill after the treatment?

By all means 'phone the acupuncturist and let him or her know. Do not blame the practitioner or the treatment because this is probably part of your own individual healing process. Be grateful that something has happened, and take your practitioner's advice about another treatment. Occasionally, people feel rotten after acupuncture because they have exceptionally unstable nervous systems. In such a case the problem will disappear after a day or two, and in the meantime your practitioner may give you a herbal remedy to help you recover.

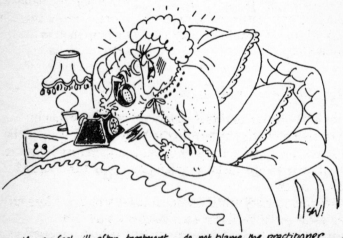

If you feel ill after treatment ... do not blame the practitioner or the treatment as this is probably part of your own individual healing process

What should I do if I think I'm not being treated properly?

This is a tricky question because it would be necessary to know why you thought you were not being treated properly. The best thing to do would be to discuss the matter with the practitioner. If, after that, you were still dissatisfied, you could discuss the matter with another practitioner to obtain an independent view.

If you have an actual complaint about your practitioner you can write to the relevant Association, but make sure your practitioner is a member first. Unless there is some specific reason to the contrary, it is a matter of courtesy to notify the practitioner concerned of your action.

Beyond all this, you have all the normal legal rights to take action against any practitioner who is guilty of malpractice. To the best of my knowledge there has never yet been such a case.

What can I do if the nearest practitioner is too far away?

If you can make one visit, the acupuncturist may be able to suggest some self-treatment at home, such as applying moxa to certain points, massaging specific points, using an electrical apparatus or doing certain types of exercises. This, of course, would depend very much upon your problem.

How does acupuncture work?

The short answer to this is that acupuncture works by correcting disharmony within the body. All the cells of the body resonate at a certain frequency, and in disease these vibrations become disharmonious. Acupuncture works by correcting this.

Acupuncturists are also among those who postulate an electromagnetic field force which surrounds and permeates the body. Disharmony in this body 'energy' and stagnation of fluids can be corrected by acupuncture.

Scientists have already shown that certain measurable effects occur after the insertion of an acupuncture needle. Some of these effects will be more closely examined in Chapter 10.

How does acupuncture stop people from smoking?

Acupuncture can help someone to stop smoking but it does not actually *stop* anyone.

It works, instead, by helping you to relax, and by improving your general vitality. This reduces the need to smoke and makes smoking more distasteful. Acupuncture also helps to clear the lungs and return them to their pristine state, thus making smoking nauseating and unpleasant.

At the same time, acupuncture helps to reduce the withdrawal effects when you stop smoking, and enables you to remain on a reasonably even keel during the difficult period which follows the cessation of any drug-taking.

Isn't it all in the mind?

The mind plays a predominant role in the cause and cure of all ills, but acupuncture only influences the mind in so far as it harmonizes the emotions and body chemistry. Acupuncture works particularly well on both children and animals where it can reasonably be assumed that there is no psychological influence.

The majority of adult patients receiving acupuncture in the West are failures of conventional medical treatment, despite the fact that it's vested with far greater authority than acupuncture.

Do I have to stop my drug treatment if I have acupuncture?

Most acupuncturists like their patients to stop any drug treatment because most drugs interfere with the treatment. However, if you are on a maintenance dose of a drug for some condition about which you are not actually consulting the acupuncturist, it may be necessary for you to remain on the drug.

It is, however, important that you notify the acupuncturist about any drugs you are taking; it would be helpful to give the exact name and the dose you have been prescribed. Sometimes, it is possible with acupuncture treatment to reduce and eventually discontinue the use of drugs, but this must be done carefully with the advice of the acupuncturist and, wherever possible, the cooperation of the prescribing doctor.

What if I want to discontinue the treatment?

There is no harm in discontinuing acupuncture treatment at any time.

Do I have to go on a diet?

You certainly do not *have* to go on a diet for acupuncture treatment to be effective, but you may be advised to make certain dietary changes. The table below gives some information about diet.

- Eat leisurely
- Do not eat when upset or tired
- Do not eat sugar
- Do not add salt to your food
- Eat only when hungry — not out of habit
- Eat more whole grains, and fresh fruit and vegetables
- Do not eat refined, manufactured or packaged foods
- Chew your food well
- Do not overeat
- Avoid deep-fried food
- Avoid coffee, tea, alcohol and chocolate
- Drink more fresh fruit juice, herb teas
- Do not eat foods you dislike
- Enhance the taste of food with herbs, spices and lemon
- Do not cook in large amounts of water
- Do not overcook. Eat plenty of raw food if possible

Some general dietary advice

Acupuncturists have always held that correct diet is important; the Chinese categorized all foods in terms of hot or cold, yang or yin, as in the following tables. This fitted in with their basic philosophy. Some acupuncturists still prescribe diets based on this teaching, but others use a more modern scientific or naturopathic approach.

Acupuncture treatment is less effective or long-lasting if there are nutritional deficiencies or other forms of dietary errors which remain uncorrected.

SOME YIN FOODS	SOME YANG FOODS
Aubergine	Carrot
Potato	Cress
Cucumber	Watercress
Mushroom	Garlic
Tomato	Onion
Spinach	Radish
Trout	Sardine
Pork	Egg
Beef	Duck
Pineapple	Apple
Orange	Strawberry
Yoghourt	Goat's milk
Sugar	Salt
Tea/coffee	Ginseng tea

Yin and yang aspects of some common foods
Yin and yang qualities are relative. For example beef, which is a yin type of meat, is more yang than apple, which is a yang type of fruit. This is because meat is more yang than fruit.

STIMULATING FOODS	CALMING FOODS	NEUTRAL FOODS
Apricot	Aubergine	Apple
Barley	Banana	French bean
Beef	Cabbage	Cauliflower
Beer	Carrot (for men)	Fig
Broad bean	Celery	Honey
Carrot (for women)	Cucumber	Papaya
Chilli	Lettuce	Peanuts
Cod	Pear	Rice
Coffee	Camomile tea	Sugar cane
Garlic	Peas	Sweet corn
Fish	Pineapple	Yoghourt
Oats	Potato	
Pepper	Pumpkin	
Shrimp	Soya beans	
Sprouts	Spinach	
	Sunflower seeds	
	Wheat	

The sedating or calming effects of some common foods

Do I need to do anything else?

Apart from judicious changes in your eating habits, you should ensure that you have enough exercise, adequate relaxation, and that you are spending some time each day in quiet meditation or cultivating the spiritual aspect of your being.

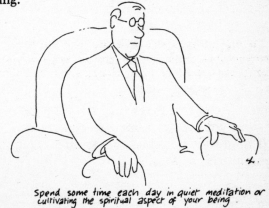

Spend some time each day in quiet meditation or cultivating the spiritual aspect of your being.

This is, perhaps, the single most important point. According to acupuncture, the really crucial part of us is not our physical bodies, but the more subtle or spiritual body which antedates, controls and determines the health of the physical body.

Cultivate good attitudes of love, acceptance, gratitude and consideration for others. This will lessen thoughts of greed, anger, jealousy, hatred, anxiety, fear and depression — all of which are very damaging to health.

Will a practitioner visit me if I am too ill to go out?

Most practitioners do visit under these circumstances, or they can refer you to someone who does.

Can the acupuncturist give me a sickness certificate?

Yes, if the practitioner is properly qualified and registered. Sickness certificates can often be written by the patient, anyway.

Can the fess be recovered from private medical insurance?

At the time of writing it is usually possible to recover acupuncture fees in this way.

Sometimes, employers will pay for the treatment of employees when they realize that the treatment will get them back to work more quickly.

If you are self-employed, you will obviously gain financially if you can carry on with your normal work sooner than you would otherwise be able to. In some cases, it might even be possible to offset acupuncture fees against tax.

Is it wise to have acupuncture for a serious problem?

Some of the conditions for which acupuncture is particularly suited and those for which it is less suited are outlined on pages 23-24.

There is no doubt that acupuncture can help in many serious conditions such as heart disease, diabetes, paralysis, mental problems, kidney disease, bronchitis, asthma and other conditions which are usually regarded as serious. Sometimes the results in these cases are quite remarkable, but it is usually necessary for the treatment to be continued for a long time and it may need to be supported by herbal therapy or homoeopathy.

Will the acupuncturist understand my condition?

Many acupuncturists are also qualified in some branch of medicine which entails their knowing western medicine. This means it is extremely unlikely that the practitioner will not have a good knowledge of your particular condition.

Of course, some people who have an unusual problem and have made a special study of it may end up knowing more about it than any doctor! Acupuncturists firmly believe that their patients do have a better understanding of their own problems than they are often given credit for, and do not think they know better than the patient about his or her own body.

Do not forget that acupuncture is often practised according to traditional concepts, in which case an acupuncture diagnosis is made. Such a diagnosis is not dependent upon any western medical knowledge. Expert acupuncturists will formulate a treatment in terms of what their own investigations reveal.

What is scientific acupuncture?

This is a type of acupuncture which is practised by those

who do not understand or do not believe in the traditional philosophy behind acupuncture. Such acupuncture is really no more scientific than traditional acupuncture, and in fact, in some cases, the treatment is the same.

So-called 'scientific acupuncture' is based on the knowledge that certain acupuncture points have specific effects. For example, a point on the top of the head is known to have a sedative action, while a point on the back of the hand between the thumb and first finger is good for controlling pain and helping with the elimination of toxins.

This type of acupuncture is used in conjunction with a western medical diagnosis, and this is another reason why it has been given the label 'scientific'. In some cases, this approach works quite satisfactorily, and occasionally may actually prove superior to the traditional methods.

In other cases, however, the traditional approach is better. It has been found by numerous authorities that the understanding of traditional philosophy is essential to the best practice of acupuncture. As traditional Chinese medicine is also behind the knowledge of scientific acupuncture, the two are so closely interwoven that in many respects they cannot be considered as separate methods.

Isn't scientific acupuncture better than traditional?

No. Traditional acupuncture has stood the test of time and has been found to work. However, that doesn't mean that it should never be changed. It can even be improved by modern medical knowledge.

Traditional Chinese medicine does not contradict western medicine, but explains things in a different way. The inclusion of precise western diagnosis and modern techniques can often help to improve the treatment and make up for some of our inadequacies such as lack of time, diminishing powers of observation and so on.

Medicine, including Chinese medicine, has always been a dynamic and developing field, and it is probably just as wrong to dismiss traditional concepts as it is to be enslaved by them.

Why is scientific acupuncture sometimes preferred?

It is really a question of diagnosis. Traditional methods of acupuncture diagnosis are always difficult, and sometimes the 'scientific' approach is more accurate. If the acupuncturist has been in practice for 40 years or more, and can spend a long time with each patient, the scientific approach would not be necessary.

In ancient China acupuncturists did a very long apprenticeship, usually with their fathers, before beginning to practise independently. Moreover, their patients' diseases were different, their vitality less affected by enervating habits, and their traditional concepts embraced a profound knowledge of medicinal herbs.

We now live in very different times, and in some cases modern medical drugs alone are enough to make the traditional type of diagnosis impossible.

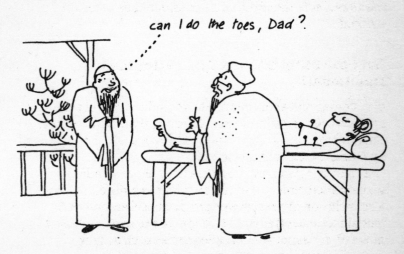

In ancient China acupuncturists did a very long apprenticeship, usually with their fathers ...

What are secondary doctor techniques?

This is the term used to describe a type of acupuncture where there is no understanding of the patient's basic disorder, and the therapist is concerned only with the relief of the symptom. This can never occur when traditional acupuncture is practised but may arise where GPs, for example, have followed a short course of purely symptomatic acupuncture. There is a real danger that such treatment will be of very limited value, without any understanding of the real purpose and healing power of acupuncture.

3.
THE MERIDIANS OF ACUPUNCTURE

'When a distinguished but elderly scientist states that something is possible, he is almost certainly right. When he states that something is impossible, he is very probably wrong.' (Clarke's First Law)

The next three chapters describe the principles on which acupuncture diagnosis and treatment are based. It is not necessary to know or understand these principles in order to benefit from acupuncture; indeed animals and young children, without any such knowledge, are frequently and successfully treated.

However, if you want to understand the theoretical basis of acupuncture, why your health problem has arisen and how acupuncture puts it right, the following chapters provide a very simplified version. The theories themselves are complex and multi-layered, and for a more detailed explanation you should consult one of the books listed on pages 117-119.

WHAT ARE MERIDIANS?

To understand how acupuncture works, it is essential to grasp the concept of meridians.

Meridians are pathways along which energy is transmitted around the body by oscillation and vibration. The meridians are sometimes called channels, but this is a slightly misleading term since their *anatomical* existence has never been demonstrated. (Although a Korean professor, Kim Bong Han, claimed to have done this some years ago, his work has not yet been fully verified.)

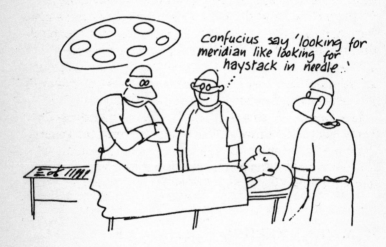

HOW DO WE KNOW THAT MERIDIANS EXIST?

The meridians have been known to the Chinese and to other traditional systems of medicine for many thousands of years. They are physiological pathways of energy, and may be demonstrated by various techniques.

Dr Nakatani from Japan was one of the first scientists to demonstrate the existence of meridians when he plotted points of low electrical resistance on the body's surface. He ended up with lines which coincided very closely with the known acupuncture meridians.

Later, Dr Reinhold Voll of the Federal Republic of Germany made similar discoveries, and also added five further meridians which had not been originally described by the Chinese! There is no unanimity of opinion among acupuncturists or scientists about the value of Voll's work, but the extent to which it has spread indicates that it provides a useful framework for a number of practitioners.

Professor Zhu Zong Xiang, who is professor of biophysics at the Department of Biophysics, Academia Sinica, Beijing, has carried out some fascinating work in which he has demonstrated the existence of meridians by what he describes as the *Propagated Sensation along the Channel* (PSC) and the *Latent Propagated Sensation along the Channel* (LPSC). His work has now become accepted throughout the world. What he describes are sensorial pathways which manifest themselves when certain points are stimulated. These pathways coincide very closely with the meridians described by the ancient Chinese.

His conclusion, as a scientist, is that the meridians do really exist. This throws into complete reverse the general trend among scientists of believing that the meridians of acupuncture and the points on the meridians are temporary manifestations with no real substance.

HOW MANY MERIDIANS ARE THERE?

In a sense there is only one single meridian which goes right round the entire body, but many different meridians are described according to their positions and functions. Five distinct groups of meridians are recognized and these are summarized in the table overleaf.

The twelve main meridians are bilateral, resulting in 24 separate pathways. Each pair is connected and related to a specific organ from which it gets its name; it is also connected to a coupled meridian and organ with which it has a special relationship. The coupled meridians each consist of a yin and a yang meridian/organ, and come under the dominance of one of the five elements.

51

TYPE OF MERIDIAN	DESCRIPTION
Main meridians (12 pairs)	Directly connected to an organ from which they get their name. Have pathways near the surface and sensitive points (acupores)
Eight extra meridians	Act as reservoirs for the main meridians. Only two have their own points
'Lo' or connecting meridians	Join each main meridian to its paired meridian
Muscle meridians	Closer to the surface than the main meridians. Feed muscles and joints
Divergent meridians	These meridians diverge from the main meridians and carry energy that will help the organs to fight off harmful influences

The five groups of meridians in acupuncture

All meridians either start or end at the hands or feet. In addition to the coupling just mentioned, the meridians can also be grouped according to the quality of energy they conduct. This also produces six pairs of meridians, each pair having one on the arm and one on the leg. These are known as the six chiaos.

To the Chinese the function of an organ was more important than its precise anatomical description or location. This arose out of the fact that they were forbidden to dissect bodies — fortunately, since otherwise they would probably have been diverted from their more metaphysical approach and become, like us, circumscribed by the material, physical body. We would then have been deprived of a considerable body of knowledge concerning our real nature.

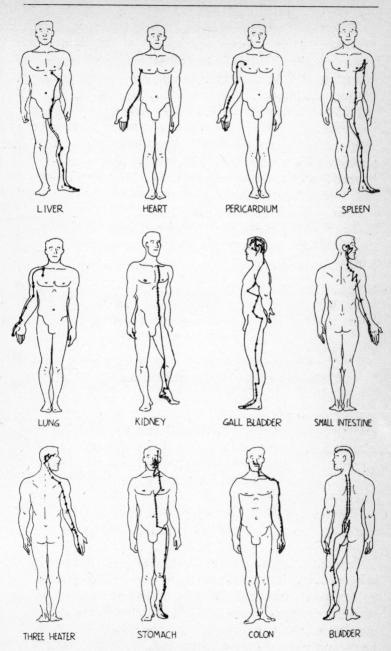

The twelve main meridians

THE ORGANS

The two tables on pages 55 and 56 list the twelve organs and summarize their functions as they were understood by the ancient Chinese.

Like everything else the organs are divided into yin and yang (see page 19). The yin organs are deeper, more solid, filled with blood and constantly active, while the yang organs are more superficial, less essential and more intermittent in their activity. These organs each influence their relevant meridian.

As an additional aid to understanding, the Chinese also likened each organ and its function to a State official. The translation of their respective duties are given in the tables.

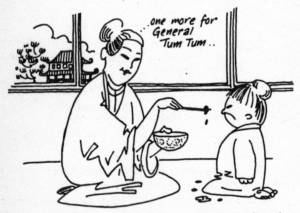

The Chinese likened each organ... to a state official.

From the table opposite it can be seen that treatment of the liver might be undertaken for a person who is unable to plan ahead, treatment of the pericardium for someone lacking in happiness, treatment of the spleen for a problem with fluid retention, and treatment of the lungs for certain types of nervous disorders. The heart, being the 'seat of the soul', might be used in a case of depression.

ORGAN	SUMMARY OF FUNCTIONS
Liver	Seat of the soul. Stores and transforms blood. (Official: general who initiates strategy)
Heart	Seat of all powers of mind and soul. (Official: ruler from whom all wisdom and insight emanate)
Pericardium	Rules the brain. Assists the heart. (Official: ambassador of happiness and joy)
Spleen	Transforms and transports fluids. (Official: guards government stores)
Lungs	Seat of the nervous system. Distribute energy (ch'i) throughout the body. (Official: administrators responsible for orderly conduct)
Kidneys	Store ch'i. Govern reproduction. (Official: secretaries of labour)

The six yin organs and their functions
The pericardium referred to in acupuncture is not an organ in the sense that we in the West would understand it. To the Chinese it was the protector of the heart, and had a strong influence on circulation and sex.

However, when we talk about treating the liver or pericardium or any other organ, what is actually meant is that acupuncture is given on specific points along the meridian related to the organ concerned. Sometimes, too, special points are treated on the bladder meridian which runs down the back, because these also relate to different organs.

ORGAN	SUMMARY OF FUNCTIONS
Gall bladder	Stores bile. Assists liver. (Official: decision-maker)
Small intestine	Receives and transforms material from stomach. (Official: executes change)
Three heater	Protector of organs. (Official: commander in chief)
Stomach	Extracts ch'i (energy) from liquids and solids. (Official: in charge of the granary)
Colon	Absorbs water and nutrients. (Official: in charge of drains and waterways)
Bladder	Stores urine. Accessory to kidney. (Official: provincial governor)

The six yang organs and their functions

The three heater is another Chinese concept, which embraces the three general processes of respiration and circulation (focused in the chest), digestion and assimilation (mainly in the upper abdomen), and elimination and sexual activity (centred in the lower abdomen). The three heater relates to all the organs and is regarded as their 'commander in chief'. It is also thought to have a special relationship with what we now know to be the endocrine system.

We can now see that a person who is unable to make decisions requires treatment of the gall bladder (meaning treatment along the gall bladder meridian, or on points which affect the gall bladder); a person who is very rigid in his or her thinking and cannot tolerate new ideas would need the small intestine treated; while a person who is unable to initiate any change might need some attention to the colon.

HEAVEN, EARTH AND HUMANS

To the Chinese heaven is yang — and the sun, in particular, is the symbol of yang; while the earth, with its comparative coolness and dampness, is yin. Humanity stands between heaven and earth, and is in a special sense a meeting point of yin and yang.

According to the great Chinese physician Ch'i Po, who laid much of the theoretical foundation of acupuncture, the human condition is composed of three parts: heaven, earth and humanity. Each of these corresponds to one of three regions, upper, middle and lower. And each region in turn has three subdivisions mirroring the three concepts of heaven, earth and humanity.

REGION	SUBDIVISION	ANATOMICAL AREA
Upper (heaven)	Heaven	Temple and brow (greater yang)
	Earth	Corner of mouth and teeth (sunlight yang)
	Humanity	Ears and eyes (lesser yang)
Middle (earth)	Heaven	Lungs (greater yin)
	Earth	Breath (sunlight yang)
	Humanity	Heart (lesser yin)
Lower (humans)	Heaven	Liver (absolute yin)
	Earth	Kidneys (lesser yin)
	Humanity	Spleen and stomach (greater yin)

The three regions and their three subdivisions, with the anatomical area to which they correspond

THE PROGRESS OF DISEASE

The understanding of these regions is important for acupuncturists because, according to tradition, disease first enters the greater yang and progresses through the different regions until it ends in absolute yin which means death.

We should not understand from this that every disease of the liver means a rapid demise: indeed we know that this is not so. Nevertheless, the progress of different diseases as outlined by Ch'i Po is interesting. If the disease is caused by cold, for example (don't forget that the Chinese were preoccupied by the pathogenic effects of the weather), it starts in the region of greater yang — so that the head and neck are in pain. On the second day, the sunlight yang receives it so that the body is feverish and the eyes ache. On the third day it penetrates the lesser yang and there is pain in the chest because the gall bladder meridian runs down the chest. In this fashion it continues through greater yin, lesser yin and finally reaches absolute yin.

GRADATIONS OF YIN AND YANG

The Chinese believed that pathways of energy connected an organ from the upper body with one from the lower body, and that these pairs of organs or meridians could be described in terms of gradations of yin or yang. They explained it like this: if you stand with your back to the sun, the area which receives the heat of the sun is greater yang. On the arm this is the area of the small intestine meridian and on the back and leg it is the bladder meridian. A little further round, on the outside of the arm and leg, are the lesser yang: the three heater and gall bladder meridians. Almost in the shade, but just able to feel the sun's warmth, is the sunlight yang: colon meridian on the arm and stomach meridian on the leg.

The figures opposite show the meridians as they are found on the body.

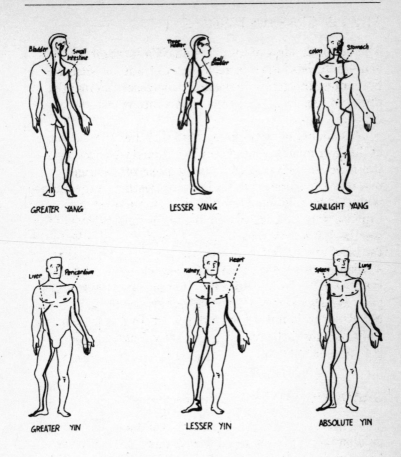

Gradations of yin and yang

SYMPTOMS

Disorders of the different organs or meridians give rise to specific symptoms. In Chinese terms the symptoms are attributed to either an excess or a deficiency of energy, but there are in fact a wide variety of disorders and degrees of disorder. Even when we talk about excess and deficiency, we can be thinking about a yang excess or deficiency or a yin excess or deficiency.

MERIDIAN/ ORGAN	SYMPTOMS
Lung	Shoulder pain, shortness of breath, phlegm, cough, cold hands and feet, dry skin, lack of energy, nervousness, hot palms, restlessness.
Colon	Frozen shoulder, constipation, diarrhoea, itchy skin, toothache, headache, sore throat, tendency to catch colds.
Stomach	Cysts in mouth, dry lips, mastitis, excess or lack of appetite, heaviness in arms and legs, swollen abdomen, yellow complexion.
Spleen	Diarrhoea, menstrual disorder, water retention, obesity, craving for sweets, cold feet, indigestion, undue fatigue.
Heart	Red complexion, palpitations, weakness of arms and legs, palms hot, swelling of nose, insomnia, excess perspiration.
Small intestine	Abdominal distension, headaches, tinnitus, poor circulation in legs, indigestion, constipation, feeling cold.
Bladder	Headache, stiff neck, back pain, nervousness, worry, anxiety, frequent urination, yawning, trembling hands.
Kidney	Breathing problems, swollen throat, joint pains, sexual disorders, restlessness, tiredness, weakness, anxiety, night sweats.
Pericardium	Palpitations, tightness of chest (angina), cold sweaty hands, absent-mindedness, fear of heights, frequent dreaming, insomnia.
Three heater	Ringing in ears, poor hearing, fatigue, indigestion, breathing problems, over-caution, urination problems.

MERIDIAN/ ORGAN	SYMPTOMS
Gall bladder	Headaches, irritability, allergy, easy bruising, eye disorders, lack of appetite, diarrhoea or constipation.
Liver	Poor appetite, tenderness in liver area, irritability, cataracts, swelling in legs, scanty yellow urine, flatulence.

The organs/meridians with some of their corresponding symptoms

THE CHINESE CLOCK

The organs in the table here are listed in a particular order. The order may at first seem strange and without any consistent pattern. In fact, however, it has been carefully chosen to follow the Chinese clock! A drawing of the clock appears overleaf.

This 'clock' is a twenty-four hour cycle which divides the day and night into two-hour periods. Each one of these is associated with a surge of energy in one of the organs and its meridians. For example, between the hours of 3 and 5 am, the lungs receive their daily booster. Following this, from 5-7 am, it is the turn of the colon.

The cycle begins with the lungs between 3 and 5 am, and for this reason it is said that these are the hours when it is most suitable to be born. This diurnal rhythm has many other implications as well, which are too complex to go into here.

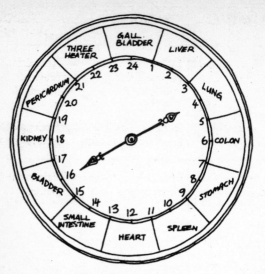

The Chinese clock

THE EIGHT EXTRA MERIDIANS

These meridians are said to be 'extra' to the main meridians. They are so powerful that they are sometimes described as the miraculous meridians. They act as reservoirs of energy and regulate the body's entire system.

Two of the extra meridians cross the centre of the body, and have their own pathways and acupuncture points; the other six share their points with some of the main meridians.

The eight extra meridians are used especially for mental problems, and are sometimes known as the psychic channels because of their power to regulate the emotions and the psyche.

The meridians referred to in the table opposite as regulators are used for the treatment of nervousness, fear, timidity, depression, apprehensiveness and bad dreams. The channels are used in cases of aggressiveness, and the vessels for strengthening the nervous system. Each is therefore associated with particular symptoms.

EXTRA MERIDIAN	FUNCTIONS	SIGNS OF DYSFUNCTION
Conception vessel (sea of all yin)	Influences lower abdomen and reproduction	Hernia, leucorrhoea, cough, menstrual disorders.
Governor vessel (sea of all yang)	Influences the back and nervous stability	Back pain, epilepsy, fever, mental disorders.
Great yin regulator (yin energy conserver)	Connects and controls all yin organs	Pain in throat, chest or genitals.
Great yang regulator (yang energy conserver)	Connects and controls all yang organs	Alternating hot and cold, boils, acne, tinnitus, toothache.
Great yin bridge channel (yin energy accelerator)	Balances yin and yang	Impotence, weak yang organs, weak legs, constipation, toxaemia in pregnancy.
Great yang bridge channel (yang energy accelerator)	Balances yin and yang	Weak yin organs, insomnia, manic-depressive state.
Belt channel (girdle channel)	Regulates physical energy of abdomen	Fullness of abdomen, weakness and motor impairment of lumbar region.
Vital vessel (penetrating channel/ vital energy regulator)	Regulates the sinews and meridians of entire body. Regulates uterus	Digestive disorders, lumbago, heart disease, gynaecological disorders.

The eight extra meridians with a summary of their functions, and the symptoms associated with them

THE TENDINO-MUSCULAR MERIDIANS

These meridians follow similar pathways to the main meridians and so are named after the same organs, but they are closer.to the surface. They contain defensive energy that will help the body to fight off harm, and this circulates in a different cycle from the ch'i (energy) in the main meridians (see page 50).

The defensive energy starts with the bladder meridian and moves on to the other yang meridians during the day and to the yin meridians at night. This explains why we tend to rub our eyes when we wake up in the morning: the bladder meridian begins at the inner corners of the eyes, and the rubbing activates the transfer from the yin of night to the yang of day.

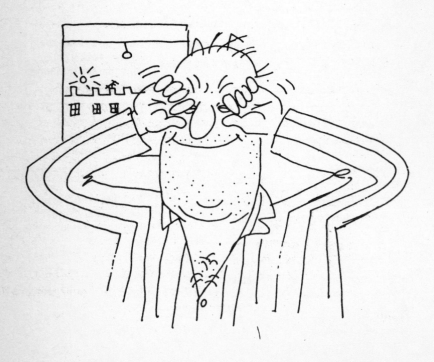

One final observation should be made about the tendino-muscular (TM) meridians: each one is more likely to show signs of disturbance during a particular month of the year, as shown in the table below. The order in which the meridians are listed corresponds to the cycle of energy in the tendino-muscular meridians.

TENDINO-MUSCULAR MERIDIAN	VULNERABLE MONTH (approx.)	TENDINO-MUSCULAR MERIDIAN	VULNERABLE MONTH (approx.)
Bladder	February	**Spleen**	August
Gall		**Lungs**	November
bladder	January		
Stomach	March	**Liver**	September
Small		**Pericardium**	October
intestine	May		
Three		**Kidney**	July
heater	June		
Colon	April	**Heart**	December

Tendino-muscular meridians and their specific months of vulnerability

DIVERGENT OR DISTINCT MERIDIANS

These meridians diverge from the main meridians. They are quite important to the acupuncturist, but need not concern us any further here.

'LO' VESSELS OR MERIDIANS

The 'lo' vessels connect together two main meridians as a pair. There are two types: transverse and longitudinal 'lo' vessels. They are both very important for the acupuncturist, and each has its own symptoms. However, they are too complex to be discussed properly here.

4.
THE FIVE ELEMENTS

'Any sufficiently advanced technology is indistinguishable from magic.' (Clarke's Third Law)

It is well known that anyone who gains power seeks to do two things in order to maintain the status quo: to promote friends (the nourishing cycle), and to remove or handicap opponents (the inhibiting cycle).

The Chinese considered that this applied, too, to the construction and working of the human body, which they represented as five 'elements' or 'phases'. These elements were wood, fire, earth, metal and water, each one of which was identified with two organs, one yang, one yin. By means of a picture, they were able to form a working model which explained the various transformations which take place within the body.

The diagram overleaf depicts these elements in their cyclical pattern, showing the 'nourishing' relationship between the various parts of the body as well as the 'inhibiting' influence which also exists between them.

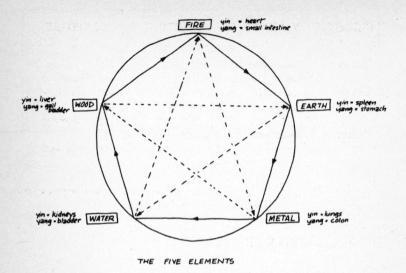

THE FIVE ELEMENTS

The nourishing cycle is depicted by a clockwise sequence (the solid line) in which each yin element is regarded as the 'mother' of the succeeding one in the circle. This is the basis of one of the great laws of acupuncture and is known as the Mother-Son Law:

MOTHER	NOURISHES	SON
Wood (liver)	fuels	fire (heart)
Fire (heart)	generates	earth or ash (spleen)
Earth (spleen)	produces	metal (lungs)
Metal (lungs)	holds	water (kidneys)
Water (kidneys)	nourishes	wood (liver)

The Mother-Son Law

Another important cycle is the inhibiting or sedating cycle (the dotted line), based on the yang organs:

ELEMENT	YANG ORGAN	ACTION	OPPOSES
Wood	(gall bladder)	covers	earth (stomach)
Fire	(small intestine)	melts	metal (colon)
Earth	(stomach)	absorbs/dams	water (bladder)
Metal	(colon)	cuts	wood (gall bladder)
Water	(bladder)	extinguishes	fire (small intestine)

The inhibiting cycle, in which an imbalance in one organ can affect the other related one

FIVE ELEMENT TREATMENT

It is already possible to see how the five elements can be used as a basis for treatment. For example, if there is a problem with the kidneys, treatment could be directed to the lungs which are the 'mother' organ. According to one theory, the problem has arisen because the vital force or ch'i is not being passed on from lungs to kidneys; by performing acupuncture on the relevant point this can be overcome.

Alternatively, if the acupuncturist found that the spleen (earth) was too strong then the spleen could be sedated. This would lift the oppressive control being exerted via the inhibiting cycle between spleen and kidneys.

It must be emphasized here that the five element approach is only one small facet of acupuncture. Some acupuncturists in the West have unfortunately exaggerated it out of all proportion.

CORRESPONDENCES

In addition, the five elements depict various phases of the bodily cycle, and each element governs a particular type of body tissue. The state of health of the 'element' and its corresponding organs may often be ascertained from the condition of the diagnostic tissue.

Another interesting application of the five elements concerns their relationship with the emotions. Anger, joy, sadness, grief and fear are all, of course, natural and necessary, but the predominance of one particular emotion or the inability to control it are signs of ill-health.

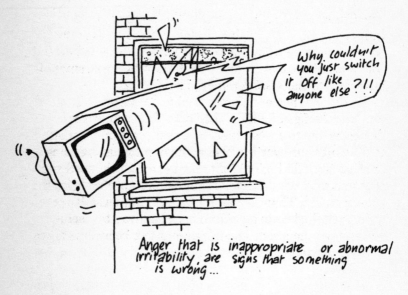

Anger that is inappropriate, or abnormal irritability, or the inability to express anger, are all signs that something is wrong — and so the liver has to be treated. Again, this is not necessarily the physical liver, but the meridian associated with the liver. Conversely, undue anger will damage the liver just as excessive excitement or joy will damage the heart, anxiety the spleen, grief the lungs and fear the kidneys. Some of these links are reflected in our own language — when we talk, for example, about someone being 'liverish' (meaning ill-tempered).

It is clear that harmful emotions are very damaging to health, and the excessive worry, anxiety and fear that predominate these days are among the most potent factors causing ill-health. We can overcome this by cultivating good positive emotions such as love, respect, trust, loyalty, serendipity and tolerance. By being less concerned about ourselves and more thoughtful of others, we do in fact unwittingly promote our own well-being.

THE WEATHER FACTOR

The Chinese also recognized that the weather could influence a person's health. Today, with all our comforts, we are insulated from the worst effects of the weather; but this was not the case in ancient China, where extremes of adverse weather were commonplace.

Traditional healers often talk about 'dampness', 'wind' and 'fire' being actually in the body. This can be very disconcerting to a westerner. However if acupuncturists talk about your liver fire blazing, they may just be using another term for high blood pressure; and if they tell you that you have wind/heat in the lungs, you probably have a common cold! There are many such phrases which are quite meaningless to a patient but which can be useful concepts to the practitioner. Ignore them, because it takes many years to learn about them!

5. MORE ABOUT TRADITIONAL IDEAS

MIDDAY — MIDNIGHT LAW

Many of the functions of our bodies are influenced by natural rhythms. It is well-known that there is a monthly cycle which affects both men and women, and is reflected in physical, mental and emotional well-being. These cycles seem to be related more to the movement of the moon than anything else but they are not synchronized; nor, for that matter, are they exactly monthly. Every so often all three will reach a pit on the same day — that's the 'off' day we all experience once in a while.

There are also rhythms that are repeated each day and night. Some hormones are secreted only at night, for example, while others mostly in the day. The Chinese recognized a 24-hour movement of energy with the Chinese clock (see page 61). The Midday-Midnight Law is based upon this biological clock.

The Chinese believed that the best time for stimulating a particular organ was at the appropriate two-hour period when its energy is 'full'. Alternatively, it should be sedated at the opposite period of the day or night. For example, the lungs should be stimulated between 3 and 5 am, and sedated between 3 and 5 pm. They were clever enough however, to think out a way to avoid seeing patients very early in the morning; they discovered that the *opposite* treatment could be applied at the opposite time on the clock. For example, instead of stimulating the lungs between 3 and 5 am, one could sedate the bladder from 3 to 5 pm. The following table may help to make this a little clearer.

TIME	ORGAN	TIME	ORGAN
3-5 am	Lungs	3-5 pm	Bladder
5-7 am	Colon	5-7 pm	Kidney
7-9 am	Stomach	7-9 pm	Pericardium
9-11 am	Spleen	9-11 pm	Three heater
11 am-1 pm	Heart	11 pm-1 am	Gall bladder
1-3 am	Small intestine	1-3 am	Liver

The Midday-Midnight Law

This establishes a special relationship between the organs in the left-hand column and those on the right. Each meridian has a special point which is used in conjunction with treatment according to the Chinese clock.

THE PULSES

The pulses are the main means of diagnosis in acupuncture. There are three pulse positions on each

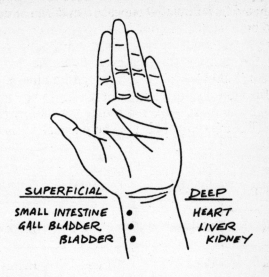

SUPERFICIAL   DEEP

SMALL INTESTINE •   HEART
GALL BLADDER   •   LIVER
BLADDER   •   KIDNEY

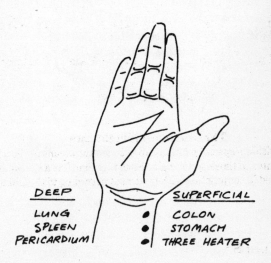

DEEP   SUPERFICIAL

LUNG   •   COLON
SPLEEN   •   STOMACH
PERICARDIUM   •   THREE HEATER

The pulses in acupuncture

wrist, and at least two levels of pulse can be felt at each point. This means that there are twelve pulses altogether, and each one reflects the state of health of one of the organs.

LEFT WRIST		RIGHT WRIST	
Superficial	**Deep**	**Deep**	**Superficial**
Small intestine Gall bladder Bladder	Heart Liver Kidney	Lungs Spleen Pericardium	Colon Stomach Three heater

The twelve pulses and their corresponding organs

HUSBAND-WIFE LAW

A relationship is believed to exist between the organs with pulses on the left wrist and those with pulses on the right. The left side is said to be the husband as the left side of the body relates to the male, while the right-sided pulse is the wife. In accordance with traditional Chinese male/female roles, the left pulses should be slightly dominant. Problems arise if the right-sided pulses are stronger than the left.

ALARM POINTS

There are points on the front of the body which often become spontaneously sensitive in acute conditions. These relate to each of the twelve organs. There are also points on the back which may become sensitive in disease. These are known as the back shu points and are often used by the acupuncturist.

Additionally, in acute conditions, other points become

tender; these are known as Ah Shi points (Chinese for 'That's it!'). Ah Shi points are not in any fixed position, but the experienced acupuncturist knows where to find them.

CHOOSING WHERE TO DIRECT TREATMENT

It can now be seen how many different organs might be involved in a condition even as straightforward as a cough. It might be the lungs, but then again it might be the colon which is the coupled organ. Or perhaps it is the spleen (the mother), or could it be the heart (the husband)? Even the bladder (the opposite organ on the 24-hour clock) might be implicated.

THE LAW OF CURE

The law of cure was promulgated by Constantine Hering, a nineteenth-century homoeopath, but it was also understood by traditional doctors long before his time. The law states that symptoms disappear:

- From interior to exterior
- From more vital to less vital
- From above downwards
- In reverse order to appearance

Because of this law of cure, symptoms which have long ago disappeared may sometimes return before final recovery. Also, problems which are internal and may be invisible and unknown, may be brought to the surface, giving the impression that things are getting worse instead of better. However, as far as the body is concerned, an unsightly and painful skin condition is safer than having toxins damaging the heart or other vital structure — even though one is visible and the other not.

One further consideration is that 'from above downwards' can be interpreted literally. On the other hand, it sometimes refers to the fact that the mental problems have to be cured before the physical symptoms will go.

6.
THE ACUPUNCTURE DIAGNOSIS

In acupuncture, just as in ordinary medicine, diagnosis is based on a large number of tests and observations. The main difference is that, in acupuncture, the diagnosis does not merely reflect the problem as it is presented, and is much more than giving a special name to a particular set of symptoms.

Sciatica, for example, is a medical diagnosis which merely gives a Greek name to what a patient may already have told the doctor in English, i.e. a pain in the leg. Moreover, it tells us nothing about the general state of health of that person, nor does it convey to anyone the type of treatment that might be indicated. Of course, a painkiller will relieve the pain. A diagnosis is not necessary for that. But, if the diagnosis was of a sacroiliac lesion, then we would know what was causing the pain in the leg and, at the same time, how best it might be treated.

The acupuncturist makes a diagnosis in terms of the body's energy (or ch'i), its blood and its fluids. These must all be harmoniously balanced and moving freely, otherwise a problem results. The acupuncturist's diagnosis is made by looking, listening (asking), touching (feeling), and examining the patient.

LOOKING

Like any doctor, most acupuncturists will look to see how you walk, stand, sit and move around. They will consider your expression and general posture, and from all this will gain a good deal of insight into what sort of person you are.

In addition, they will note a number of things which are of special interest to an acupuncturist: how you are dressed, the colour of your clothes, and any colours noticeable in your facial complexion. Later, your eyes and tongue will be examined, as will your hair, nails, ears and skin, because all these give further information about your general state of health.

LISTENING

Of course, all acupuncturists will listen to what you have to say about your problem. They will also ask a number of questions designed to pinpoint the basic problem in terms of traditional Chinese medicine. They will want to know, for example, at what time of day you feel worse or better, whether your symptoms are aggravated by heat, damp, cold or wind, whether they appear or become worse at a particular time of year or, if you are a woman, whether they are related to your monthly cycle.

More importantly, you will be asked questions about your emotional state. Are you quick to anger? Are you sad? Are you lacking in spirit or *joie de vivre*? Do you have rapid mood swings or are you a habitual worrier?

At the same time the acupuncturist will be listening to the sound of your voice, since a lot can be learned even from that.

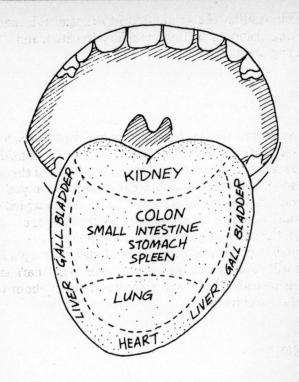

Each area of the tongue is considered to be related to a particular organ

FEELING

Acupuncturists will feel or palpate any area of the body about which you are complaining, but they will also feel areas or points on the skin quite a distance away from the problem that brought you to them. In particular, they will press lightly on the alarm points and other points (see pages 76-77) to discover whether they are tender.

Your abdomen may be palpated, as may various points on your feet. And of course, and very important, the twelve pulses which were described earlier will be taken.

EXAMINATION

Apart from palpating various areas, acupuncturists will examine any joints which might be stiff or painful. They will carry out a normal range of tests which are applicable to a given situation, and these may include the familiar reflex tests.

Some acupuncturists take routine blood-pressure readings, and some carry out basic urine analysis. Others practise what is known as bioenergetic medicine, which means that they use instruments to find some of the points which they might otherwise have palpated with their fingers. The instruments give a reading which, if abnormal, can be corrected by treatment.

Many acupuncturists use the technique of applied kinesiology. This consists of testing various muscles to obtain a picture of the state of energy in the different organs. These are illustrated in the figure below.

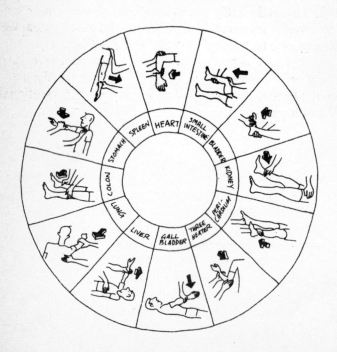

Applied kinesiology, however, can also be used for a wide range of investigations, by looking for a change in muscle response when a particular point on the body is touched. First of all, a muscle is tested — and, for convenience, one of the muscles which move the arm is usually selected. The examiner then moves the arm in a direction which opposes the muscle being tested and at the same time asks the patient to 'hold'. Provided the muscle is functioning correctly, the patient will be able to lock the arm in position as long as undue force or sudden movement are avoided.

The examiner now touches the relevant point. This could be a pulse, an alarm point or any one of a large number of points on the body. If there is an abnormality or a need for treatment at that particular point, there will be a change in the function of the muscle being tested.

This relatively new technique was originally discovered by Dr G. Goodheart in the USA, in around 1960: so it was not understood by the ancient Chinese. There are many things we can do today which the Chinese were not aware of. Whereas they excelled in patience and observation, we can offer new techniques and technology. These techniques and technological advancements, however, are of therapeutic value only in so far as they are consistent with the fundamental laws of acupuncture and traditional Chinese medicine.

7.
FORMULATING THE TREATMENT

CHOOSING THE POINTS FOR ACUPUNCTURE

Local and distal points

To treat a patient the acupuncturist may choose to use a combination of acupuncture points in the area of the problem, coupled with points near the opposite end of the meridian concerned (called 'distal' points). This often helps to reinforce the action at the site of the problem.

In addition there are special distal points which influence particular areas of the body.

The influential points

Respiratory tissue, bone and cartilage, blood, internal organs, the circulatory system, muscles and tendons and bone marrow all have influential points. Where indicated, these points may be used in conjunction with other points. In asthma, for example, the distal point for the lungs and

LOCATION	AREA OF INFLUENCE
On the hand	Face. Front of head
On the wrist	Back of head and neck. Back of chest and lungs
On the lower arm	Front of chest. Upper abdomen
Below the knee	Lower abdomen and organs
The back of the knee	Lower back. Urinogenital organs
On the lower leg	Pelvic organs and external genitalia

Principal distal points and their spheres of influence

the influential point for the solid organs might be combined.

The Chinese clock

A special point on each main meridian is termed the horary point. This may be used to stimulate the meridian at its appropriate time on the Chinese clock (see pages 61-62). Alternatively, the same point may be used at the opposite period of the 24-hour clock to sedate the meridian. For example, the stomach may be stimulated between 7 and 9 am, or sedated between 7 and 9 pm.

Symptomatic points

Some points are known to be effective for treating specific symptoms. For asthma, for example, there are two points on the back which are actually called 'soothing asthma points'. Another point at the top of the breast bone is also helpful in an acute asthmatic attack. And, finally, each meridian has one xi (pronounced 'shi') cleft point which is useful for acute conditions. In the case of asthma, treatment could well be applied to the xi cleft point on the lung meridian.

Front mu and back shu points

The combination of the alarm points (front mu points) and back associated points (shu points) constitute a useful form of treatment in many cases.

Homeostatic points

These are points which are particularly helpful in restoring balance and harmony to the body.

Immune enhancing points

These points are particularly useful if there is any kind of infection.

Sedative points

Are specially useful for reducing anxiety. Consequently, they may be used for virtually any disease.

Ah shi points

Are useful in acute disorders. (See page 77.)

Nose acupuncture

There are points on the nose which relate to all parts of the body. These, however, are less often used than the acupuncture points on the ear, described overleaf.

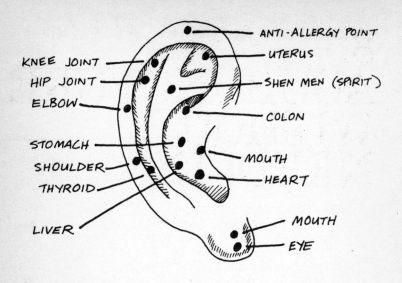

Ear acupuncture

There are points on the external ear which relate to every part of the body. These points may be used by themselves or in combination with other points.

Head or scalp needling

Is a recent innovation. Points are selected on the head which relate to different areas of the brain. They are often useful for paralysis and disorders of sensation.

8. ACUPUNCTURE WITHOUT NEEDLES

MOXIBUSTION

Moxibustion is the treatment of acupuncture points by heat. It has always formed an integral part of traditional acupuncture, and is particularly useful in cases where the ch'i (energy) or the blood has accumulated and is not moving properly.

It is also used where there is a deficiency of yang or an excess of yin, and where disease results from the invasion of cold. It is particularly helpful for chronic conditions.

Moxibustion involves burning 'moxa', usually the dried leaves of a herb called mugwort. It may be done in the following ways: burning a moxa stick near the acupuncture point; burning a small amount of moxa on the point itself; burning a larger amount of moxa on a slice of garlic or ginger; burning moxa wrapped around the needle head; burning a chunk of moxa stick on the needle; using a stimulator to impart heat to the point.

Strictly speaking, moxa is not an alternative to needle

treatment, and is a complementary form of 'acupuncture' which dates back to the Stone Age. No qualified acupuncturist would practise without including moxa treatment, in cases where it is needed.

Conditions where moxibustion is usually beneficial include:

bronchitis	diverticulitis	paralysis
pneumonia	urinogenital disorders	lumbago
asthma	constipation	arthritis
gastric problems	haemorrhoids	incontinence
diarrhoea	fluid retention	spinal deformity
appendicitis		

One of the most remarkable uses of moxibustion is on a point on the little toe to bring about movement of the foetus during pregnancy. For this reason it is employed to turn a malpositioned foetus.

CUPPING

This is another traditional treatment which has always been considered as a complement to acupuncture. It involves taking small glass cups, burning a small amount of cotton wool impregnated with alcohol for a few seconds inside the cup, and then placing the cup over the area to be treated. A vacuum will be created inside the cup, and this causes the underlying flesh to be sucked up.

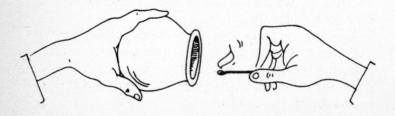

In earlier times the cups were made from animals' horns, and the vacuum was created by sucking the air out and plugging the hole. Later cups were made of bamboo, earthenware, copper and iron.

Cupping is particularly beneficial for asthma, bronchitis, lumbago, headaches and rheumatism.

SOME MODERN TECHNIQUES

Electrical stimulation

This is a modern technique which was not, of course, used by the ancient Chinese.

Electrical stimulation of the needles, once they have been inserted, is very useful in many painful conditions, and is particularly helpful when acupuncture is being used to produce analgesia during surgery. Electrical stimulation may also be done directly on the acupoints, thus avoiding the need for needles.

Sensitive electrical apparatus can help to detect acupuncture points, making it very useful in ear acupuncture, where the points are so close together.

Treatment by laser

Laser is a special kind of light which has only one wavelength and does not spread out like ordinary light. Scientists term this coherence, and it is a characteristic that makes laser light very useful in acupuncture. Of course acupuncturists don't use powerful lasers, any more than they connect people to the mains to give them electrical treatment. The lasers used in acupuncture are very weak and entirely safe.

This bears out a general physiological rule which states that minute doses of a drug are stimulating, moderate doses first stimulate, then depress, while large doses produce brief stimulation followed by strong inhibitory effects which may be fatal.

The laser has been shown to be as effective as needles in stimulating acupuncture points for most conditions. It has the advantage that it is entirely painless and carries no possible risk of infection.

Sound

Both sound waves and ultrasound have been used to stimulate acupuncture points, and the results have been found to be satisfactory. It seems that acupuncture points are capable of extracting the energy from almost any source, whether heat, light, sound, magnetism, electricity or radio waves. The absorbed energy is then changed into what is required by the body, and what is not needed is presumably discarded.

Magnetism

We know comparatively little about the effects of magnetism on living organisms except that North Pole magnetism seems to sedate biological functioning, while South Pole magnetism seems to promote or accelerate it. North Pole magnetism is therefore useful for tumours or active infections, whereas South Pole magnetism is indicated in cases of pain or paralysis.

The application of magnetism to acupuncture points is still in its infancy but may prove to be a valuable technique in the future.

Shortwave and microwave

These are both now standard treatments in physiotherapy, but their application to acupuncture points is experimental.

HOT NEEDLE

This is a special technique, different from the application

of moxa upon a needle (see page 89). In the case of the hot needle, a special needle is brought to red heat and plunged for a fraction of a second into the tissue. It has been used effectively for ganglions and some kinds of thyroid swellings (goitres).

MASSAGE

This is a traditional accompaniment to acupuncture. It should really be considered as complementary rather than an alternative.

The acupuncture points themselves are massaged either by pressing with the thumb or fingers (sometimes known as 'shiatsu'), or by making small circles around the point with a finger tip. A clockwise movement is said to sedate the point, while an anti-clockwise motion stimulates it.

One of the great advantages of massage is that it is not limited to acupuncture points. Since it involves the transfer of therapeutic energy, it can be of enormous additional benefit.

HOMOEOPUNCTURE

This judicious combination of acupuncture and homoeopathy has been developed in Sri Lanka under the guidance of Professor Anton Jayasuriya.

Once a homoeopathic remedy has been correctly selected for a patient, the acupuncture needle is dipped into the liquid remedy and then used to puncture the acupoint. Because homoeopathy works with minute doses, this method of administration has been found to be particularly advantageous as it eliminates all the problems associated with oral homoeopathic medication.

For example, homoeopathic remedies should not be taken orally for two or three hours after a meal, nor for half an hour beforehand. You cannot even clean your teeth after a dose of a homoeopathic drug. The drug itself is rendered useless if exposed to strong odours or scents, and its effects are said to be neutralized by coffee or a hot bath.

When given with acupuncture, all these problems are overcome. Moreover, the aggravation which is often associated with good homoeopathic prescribing is minimized or prevented.

Homoeopuncture has been found to be very useful in childbirth for the relief of pain, and it has also been given very successfully in pre-operative and post-operative care.

SELF-TREATMENT

There are numerous books which deal with acupuncture without needles. These books usually refer to massaging acupuncture points, and give lengthy descriptions of how to treat yourself in this way. There is no reason at all why anyone should not do this, provided that there is no serious health problem involved. If in any doubt, it is wise to check with your GP or an acupuncturist.

Instruments designed to deliver electric stimulation are also available for self-treatment. Before purchasing such equipment, it might be advisable to check on its safety and usefulness with one of the official organizations listed on pages 111-112.

9. SOME PARTICULAR USES

CHILDBIRTH

One of the more interesting applications of acupuncture is in labour and childbirth. It can be used to regulate the later stages of pregnancy as well as to encourage a satisfactory labour and healthy birth.

More importantly, it can be used to reduce the pains of childbirth. This is of great benefit to the child as it avoids the need for hazardous drugs.

LACK OF ENERGY

This is one of the most common symptoms. In the USA it is the single most usual reason why people consult their doctors. However, conventional medicine can offer very little help, while acupuncture is frequently used with great success.

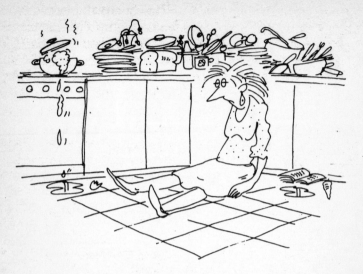

Acupuncture is frequently used for patients who suffer from lack of energy.

SMOKING

Acupuncture has a good track record for helping people to give up smoking (see also page 40).

ENURESIS

This is one of many behavioural problems that often responds well to acupuncture.

SURGERY

Acupuncture can be used to produce analgesia, enabling surgery to be undertaken without any conventional anaesthetic. Now it is seldom used in this way, however, as most patients would prefer not to be conscious during an operation (and surgeons prefer an unconscious patient too!).

Acupuncture is very useful in cases where urgent surgery needs to be done on someone who, for example, is anaemic, and cannot safely undergo surgery in the usual way. Such cases are uncommon in the West but do occur in Third World countries. Acupuncture is also useful in dentistry, but would normally only be used for patients who are allergic to chemical analgesics.

DRUG ADDICTION

The principle of treatment in drug addiction is similar to that of giving up smoking, but the treatment usually has to be much more frequent and for longer periods of time. In severe cases it may be necessary in the early stages for the addict to have as many as three treatments a day, each lasting for an hour or more.

Another important effect of acupuncture is to help restore the body's own opiate production which the drugs often suppress. Hence, acupuncture is effective in preventing many of the physical withdrawal symptoms.

The treatment can be very helpful but usually needs to be carried out in a special purpose-designed unit.

CANCER

In all serious and chronic conditions such as cancer, multiple sclerosis, Parkinsonism, heart disease and diabetes, acupuncture can often contribute towards recovery, but it usually needs to be combined with other treatments. Dietary regulation and nutritional supplements are almost always also necessary.

FUNCTIONAL DISORDERS

It is for the common, less serious functional disorders
(which can often completely upset a person's life) that
acupuncture can be most helpful, often dramatically so.

Conditions such as migraine, headaches, sinusitis,
anxiety, tension, sleeping difficulties, sexual problems,
menstrual disorders, constipation, diarrhoea, nausea and
musculoskeletal pains are often relieved by just two or
three acupuncture sessions. Once the symptoms have been
cleared, it is important to have further check-ups at
regular intervals.

AIDS

Several medical doctors are successfully treating AIDS
with acupuncture.

There is, incidentally, no need to worry at all about the
risk of contracting AIDS from acupuncture needles —
provided you attend a properly qualified acupuncturist.

You are not allowed to give blood after acupuncture
treatment, to safeguard the blood transfusion service from
anyone who might have been to an unqualified
practitioner.

10.
HOW DOES ACUPUNCTURE WORK?

'The only way of discovering the limits of the possible is to venture a little way past them into the impossible' (Clarke's Second Law)

In the end we always come back to the same question, usually asked at the beginning: 'How does acupuncture work?'.

The reason the answer to this question is difficult to grasp is that, in acupuncture, we are confronted by a new reality which our minds are not conditioned to accept. If you gave an apple pip to someone who knew nothing at all about agriculture and who had never seen any seeds or pips before, and you told that person that you were going to plant it in the ground and that later it would grow and become a tree, he or she might scarcely believe you. You might be able to answer the question 'How does it happen?' by talking about genes or chromosomes, or RNA or DNA. But even if you were a molecular biologist, you would have to admit, in the end, that you did not really know.

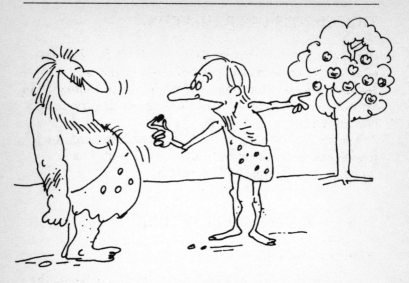

We cannot say why that apple pip knows how to grow into an apple tree and not into a daffodil or an oak tree. We do not know exactly why it does not rot in the ground like a leaf or the rest of the fruit. We do not know how it can survive the ravages of the soil and actually convert the contents of the soil into its own structure. Still less can we understand how it is able to become an apple tree.

Our difficulty in understanding how acupuncture works is on a similar scale. We know that the living organism is surrounded by cosmic energy which it absorbs, transmutes and uses for its own ends. We can say that acupuncture restores or improves that process when things have gone wrong. That explains why animals can be successfully treated by acupuncture — even plants are amenable to treatment. We may never know or fully understand exactly how acupuncture works. That it does work is beyond doubt.

If we can shake off the shackles of materialism and begin to see with the eyes of a child those things which are not visible, we will have set out on the journey towards comprehending the reality of the universe and how the human body really works. And, at that stage, we will no longer need to ask: 'How does acupuncture work?'

THE SCIENTIFIC EXPLANATION

Once scientists saw that acupuncture did in fact have an effect which could no longer be denied or ignored, it became necessary for them to 'explain' the phenomenon in terms which were consistent with their existing framework of knowledge.

The fact is that acupuncture does not fit well into such a model, and so far the scientific theories about it have failed to come to grips with the reality.

THE EFFECTS OF ACUPUNCTURE

Analgesic effect

Science has however, to a very large extent, explained the mechanisms by which acupuncture can relieve pain. The best-known theories about this are the *gate control theory* and the *endorphin theory*. The gate control theory postulates a functional 'gate' which closes against the

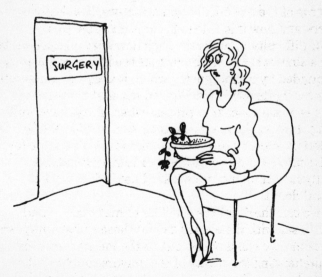

Even plants are amenable to acupuncture treatment...

nerve impulses which are interpreted as pain. The endorphin theory claims that morphine-like substances are released in the body under acupuncture treatment. These morphine-like substances are called endorphins because they are made within the body itself, and are the body's own painkillers.

Homoeostatic effect

This describes the ability of acupuncture to bring about physiological regulation and harmony. It has now been shown that acupuncture is able to regulate blood pressure, heart rate, urinary excretion, respiration, temperature, ionic balance and endocrine functioning. This normalizing process is probably the most important function of acupuncture. Science has now demonstrated that it takes place, but has so far failed to explain how.

Immune-enhancing effect

Another action of acupuncture strengthens the body's resistance to disease. Physiological measurement before and after acupuncture has demonstrated that it brings about a change in the concentration of white blood cells, opsonins, kinins and antibodies — all of which contribute to immunity. However, science has been unable to explain how these changes are brought about.

Psychological effect

Acupuncture has also been proved to have a calming or tranquillizing action. This is thought to be the result of changes in certain chemicals around the brain such as dopamine. These changes have been measured, but not explained.

Sedative effect

Investigations have clearly shown that there are changes

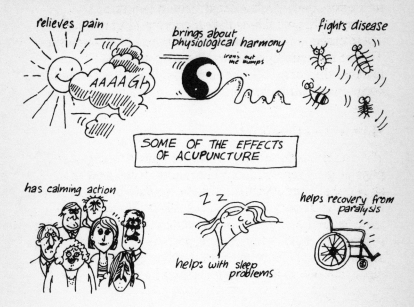

in brain activity after acupuncture. A decrease in delta and theta waves has been noted on electroencephalograms during acupuncture, and this could very well be the reason why it is helpful in sleep disturbances, anxiety states, phobias, addictions, epilepsy and behavioural problems.

Motor recovery effect

Patients who have become paralyzed for one reason or another have sometimes recovered after acupuncture treatment.

CONCLUSION

There are many scientific theories about the effects of acupuncture, but none has yet satisfactorily explained how it works. Until that explanation arrives, we continue to use the traditional Chinese explanation. No better summary of this can be found than in Professor Jayasuriya's book *Clinical Acupuncture*: 'Even though many theories are now current, the secret of acupuncture will not be easily solved. As it is a very complex phenomenon, it will remain a mystery inside, an enigma, surrounded by total darkness for many more decades to come.'

HOW TO FIND A PRACTITIONER

The registers below will provide a list of qualified practioners on request. All are the members of the British Acupuncture Council. Please note that associations offering lists of practioners usually request a stamped addressed envelope and often a small fee.

British Acupuncture Council
Park House
206 Latimer Road
London, W10 6RE
Tel: 0181 - 964 0222
The British Acupuncture Council was formed in 1995 by the unification of five member groups of The Council for Acupuncture. It was unanimously agreed that one body should represent and govern professionally qualified traditional acupuncturists in all aspects of their work.
Members are bound by the Council's Code of Ethics and Practice. An information leaflet is available on request.

British Acupuncture Accreditation Board

Park House
206 Latimer Road
London
W10 6RE
Tel: 0181 - 968 3469
An independant body monitoring the training of
acupuncturists. Information is available directly
from the above address.

The British Acupuncture Association

34 Alderney Street
London SW1V 4EU
Longest established acupuncture association in the
UK with a reputation for excellance throughout the
world, including the People's Republic of China.
Members are all qualified in some form of medicine
in addition to accupuncture.
Publications include a yearbook.
Members use the letters MBAcA, or FBAcA.

The British College of Acupuncture

8 Hunter Street
London WC1N 1BN
Tel: 0171 - 833 8164
At present only postgraduate courses are offered and
lead to licentiate diploma in acupuncture, and after
the advanced course membership of the college.
The college also has a teaching clinic.
Tel: 0171 - 837 6429.

The International College of Oriental Medicine UK Ltd.
Green Hedges House
Green Hedges Avenue
East Grinstead
West Sussex RH19 1DZ
Tel: 01342 - 313106
Founded in 1972, the college offers a 4-year full-time course and part-time courses leading to licentiate.
Short courses in Swedish massage are also available.
The college's teaching clinic is at the same address.

London School of Acupuncture & Traditional Chinese Medicine
60 Bunhill Row
London
EC1Y 8QD
Tel: 0171 - 490 0513
Offers a full-time B.Sc., Hons., in traditional Chinese medicine and acupuncture validated by Westminster University. Postgraduate diploma in Chinese Herbal Medicine courses are to professional entry with clinical observation and practice throughout. The school maintains close links with colleges in the People's Republic of China.

College of Traditional Acupuncture
Tao House
Queensway
Leamington Spa
Warwickshire CV31 3LZ
Tel: 01926 - 422121
Offers part-time courses leading to licentiate in acupuncture and an extensive programme of post-graduate studies.
Weekend-based courses are available in Leamington Spa or Glasgow Tel: 0141 - 424 4800.
The college's teaching clinic is at the same address.

Acupuncture is widely practised around the world, and many countries have their own associations and registers. Information about acupuncture and local practioners can also be obtained from:

CANADA

Canada Acupuncture Foundation
Suite 302
7321 Victoria Park Avenue
Markham
Ontario L3R 2Z8

Mrs Doris Sweetnam
PO Box 3
Stittsville
Ontario K0A 3G0
Tel: (613) 836 3005

AUSTRALIA

Brisbane College of Traditional Acupuncture
2nd floor, Century House
316 Adelaide Street
Brisbane 4000
Queensland

Acupuncture Association of Victoria
126 Union Road
Surry Hills
Victoria 3127

Acupuncture College of Australia
520 Harris Street
Ultimo
Sydney, NSW

NEW ZEALAND

A.T. Bryant
1-38 Jutland Road
Tabapuna

Miss A. Bong
43 Mellons Bay road
Howick
Auckland
Tel: (9) 534 3764

FURTHER INFORMATION

The Institute for Complementary Medicine
The Information Officer
PO Box 194
London
SE16 1QZ
Tel: 0171 - 237 5165
An independant charity which runs an information service (including listings of practitioners) for the public, media and professionals. Publishes a journal and a yearbook.

AcuMedic Centre
101-105 Camden High Street
London NW1 7JN
Tel: 0171 - 388 5783
An independant information centre on many aspects of Chinese medicine including associations, equipment, seminars etc. The clinic has a profes-sional dispensary service for Chinese herbalists and

practitioners, together with 7 doctors and specialists. Also offers a good selection of books.

Community Health Foundation
188 Old Street
London EC1V 9BP
Tel: 0171 - 251 4076
Provides information and facilities at all levels for the teaching and practical application for preventive medicine.
Has a bookshop.
Emphasizes shiatsu rather than acupuncture.

Natural Health Clinic Network
4 Hardwick Road
Ryegate
RH2 9HT
Tel: 01737 - 217 555
An association of natural health centres and individuals who support a number of common aims. These are to provide information and guidance on the nature and availability of natural therapies, to educate in the promotion of health and the prevention of ill-health through self-care and self-responsibility, and to encourage co-operation between practitioners of natural therapies and orthodox medicine.

GLOSSARY

AIDS — Acquired Immune Deficiency Syndrome. This is
a collapse of the immune system owing to poor nutrition
and exposure to the virus concerned. The virus is not
easily transmitted, but may be passed on by injections or
sexual intercourse

Alarm points — A specific set of points on the front of the
body which frequently reflect the state of their
corresponding meridians by becoming spontaneously
tender when there is a disorder. Many other similar points
exist including 'ah shi' points and 'shu' points

Allopathic — Describes the basis of modern 'scientific' or
Western medicine. The word means treatment with
opposites (hence the use of anti-inflammatory drugs to
bring down inflammation, analgesics to dull pain,
antibiotics to control bacteria, etc.)

Ah shi points — Points or tiny areas on the surface of the body which become spontaneously sensitive when there is a disorder. Their positions vary according to what is wrong

Ch'i — Oriental term pronounced 'chee' in Chinese or 'key' in Japanese. It describes the energy or force which protects, restores, motivates and vitalizes the body

Chinese clock — The 24-hour cyclic ebb and flow of body energy in each of the meridians

Distal points — Points lying on the meridians below the elbow or knee, which may be used when the opposite end of the meridian is either being treated or lies within an area of dysfunction

Homoeopathy — System of medicine based on the theory that 'like cures like'. Patients with a set of symptoms receive drugs which are themselves capable of producing similar symptoms. The remedies are extremely dilute and probably work because of a vibration set up in the diluent

Homoeopuncture — A careful and judicious combination of homoeopathy and acupuncture in which the acupuncture needle is dipped into the appropriate homoeopathic remedy before being introduced into the patient. Since only tiny amounts of homoeopathic remedies are required, this is an excellent way of administering them

Hormones — Chemicals secreted in the body which act as messengers to regulate most body activities

Laser — (Acronym for Light Amplification by Stimulated Emission of Radiation). A device which produces a beam of light of a single wavelength (monochromatic). Being coherent, it can be projected a long distance without being dispersed. In acupuncture a very weak laser is used to treat an acupuncture point

Meridian — Line of transmission of vital energy and 'blood' which crosses the entire body. This line or channel is subdivided into many portions with various names and functions

Neuralgia — Inflammation of a nerve causing a throbbing or gripping pain

Pericardium — In Western medicine the pericardium is the membrane which encases the heart, but in Chinese medicine it refers to a range of functions connected with augmenting the heart, circulation and sexual activity. Sometimes called 'heart constrictor' (because it has a controlling function over the heart) or 'circulation sex'

Phobias — Irrational fears

Shiatsu — Japanese term meaning massage by pressing with the tip of the thumb or finger. Pressure is applied mainly to acupuncture points, but may also be done all over the body

Shu points — A series of points found on the bladder meridian on the back. Each one relates to a corresponding organ in the body. They may become spontaneously tender and the organs may be affected by treating them

Tao — The unknowable and ultimate cause which expressed itself by the polar forces of yin and yang bringing about creation. All things must be in conformity with the Tao and the inherent laws of the universe. By disobeying these laws, people sow the seeds of disharmony and disease

Three heater — The three heater represents the three 'burning spaces' in the body where metabolism is chiefly centred: the chest, upper abdomen, and lower abdomen. In the chest it relates to respiration and circulation, in the upper abdomen to digestion and assimilation, and in the lower abdomen to sexual activity and elimination. Also known as the 'triple burner', 'triple metabolism' or 'body cavity'

Tinnitus — A ringing or rushing noise heard in one or both ears when there is no actual source of such noise. It may be continuous or intermittent

Xi-cleft point — On every meridian there is one point known as the xi-cleft or accumulation point. Its chief use is in acute conditions affecting the meridian or its related organ

Yang — The principle found throughout the universe of warmth, activity, life, dryness, maleness and superficiality

Yin — The principle found throughout the universe of cold, structure, immobility, dampness, femaleness and depth. Neither yin nor yang can exist alone

READING LIST

The following is a selection from the books available on acupuncture and Chinese medicine:

Acupuncture: How it Works and How it is Used Today, by F. Mann (Pan, 1985)
More difficult to understand than most of the books recommended here. It does, however, give a fairly comprehensive view of the subject.

The Chinese Art of Healing, by S. Palos (Bantam Books, 1971)
This is an extremely good book and gives a great deal of information while remaining accessible to the general reader.

The Healing Power of Acupuncture, by Michael Nightingale (Javelin Books, 1986)
This book is easily read, yet full of information, and would make an extremely good follow-up book to this one.

Modern Chinese Acupuncture, by G.T. and N.R. Lewith
(Thorsons, 1980)
Fairly technical and more suitable for professionals.

Acupuncture, The Chinese Art of Healing, by M. Duke
(Constable, 1973)
Very informative basic book on acupuncture which gives a
good insight into traditional Chinese medicine, including
herbal practice. Well illustrated.

Clinical Acupuncture, by A. Jayasuriya (Acupuncture
Foundation of Sri Lanka, 1985)
Though expensive and written for the student or
practitioner, this book is well worth reading by anyone
who wants to make a serious study of acupuncture.
Probably the best basic book on clinical acupuncture in
print.

The Principles and Practice of Moxibustion, by R.
Newman Turner and R.H. Low (Thorsons, 1981)
This well-illustrated book on moxibustion was the first in
English, and is something of a classic. Although written for
the practitioner, it is quite readable by the non-specialist.
More technical material is confined to tables.

The Yellow Emperor's Classic of Internal Medicine, trans.
by Ilza Veith (University of California Press, 1965)
This translation of the earliest book on acupuncture is a
must for anyone who seriously wishes to study the subject.

Harmony Rules, by G. Butt and F. Bloomfield (Arrow
Books, 1985)
Mainly concerned with nutrition from the point of view of
Chinese medicine, but also explains a good deal of the
traditional thinking which forms the backdrop to
acupuncture.

The Taoist Way of Healing, by Chee Soo (Aquarian Press, 1986)
Says very little about acupuncture itself, but illustrates how it is only one part of a whole system of healing, with the same unifying philosophy.

Modern Chinese Acupuncture, by G.T. and N.R. Lewith (Thorsons, 1986)
A short, basic textbook on acupuncture. Though aimed at doctors, it is also reasonably easy to follow. Good follow-up reading. The prescriptive part of the book is decidedly medical rather than traditional.

Acupuncture Energy in Health and Disease, by H. Woollerton and J. McLean (Thorsons, 1979)
Intended for the more advanced student of acupuncture, it gives a fairly detailed account of the formation of energies within the body and how they can be used in acupuncture treatment.

Japanese Acupuncture, by M. Hashimoto (Liveright, 1971)
A simple little book on acupuncture which is quite easy to read.

First Aid at Your Fingertips, by D. and J. Lawson-Wood (Health Science Press, 1976)
Short book illustrating the points for first-aid treatment.

The Complete Book of Acupuncture, by S.T. Chang (Celestial Arts, 1976)
Very comprehensive book on basic acupuncture. Highly recommended for follow-up reading as it is packed with information and reasonably easy to follow.

INDEX

COLOUR HEALING

A practical guide to understanding the healing power of colour

LILIAN VERNER BONDS

Why do you love some colours and hate others? Why does the colour of a room have an effect on your mood? Colour surrounds and affects everyone, and by fostering a greater awareness of the language and psychology of colour, we can learn to appreciate, understand and use it in every area of our lives.

This fascinating and life-enhancing book will give you a simple understanding of the nature of colour, and show you how to use colour for personal growth and healing by applying a spectrum of practical techniques, from interior design and choosing what colours to wear, to eating and drinking coloured foods!

MEDITATION

A practical introduction to the technique and its benefits

ERICA SMITH and NICK WILKS

People of any age, condition and circumstance can meditate, and as a result of regular practice, most people quite naturally begin to adopt a healthier way of life. It can benefit those suffering from stress and anxiety, and improve emotional well-being in everyone.

The first two chapters of this informative and enlightening guide explain what meditation is and how it can help you. The rest of the book provides practical information about how to practice it, A wide range of techniques is described and the questions most commonly asked about meditation are answered. Advice is given on meditating at home and choosing a teacher, and the reference section at the end of the book lists a number of teachers and organisations who give instruction in meditation.

FLOWER REMEDIES

An introduction to over 200 international flower remedies, their benefits and uses.

PETER MANSFIELD

Flower remedies are a wonderfully simple and totally safe way of helping the body to fulfill its natural tendency to be healthy. Working on an emotional level, these remedies have the effect of making you 'feel better'. They stimulate the body to overcome the causes of physical illnesses and recover its equilibrium. In this way the remedies also complement other traditional or alternative healing methods.

HYPNOTHERAPY

A practical guide to improving health and well being with hypnosis

URSULA MARKHAM

Hypnotherapy is increasingly being used to relieve and cure a wide range of disorders, and is becoming a recognised and established therapy within the medical profession. Many sufferers are, however, deterred from seeking help because of fear or ignorance about how hypnosis and hypnotherapy work.

This book will set the record straight. It explains exactly what hypnosis is, and describes how it can bring great benefit in overcoming a vast number of problems; phobias, smoking, exam pressure, over eating or even general stress. The book covers what to expect from your first and subsequent consultations, and how relaxation and visualisation can be practised at home. Further information is given on how to find out more, and where to find a therapist.

To order your copy direct from Vermilion, use the form below or call TBS DIRECT on **01621 819596**.

Please send me

......copies of **COLOUR HEALING** @ £7.99 each
......copies of **MEDITATION** @ £6.99 each
......copies of **FLOWER REMEDIES** @ £7.99 each
......copies of **HYPNOTHERAPY** @ £6.99 each

Mr/Ms/Mrs/Miss/Other (Block Letters)

....

Address..

....

....

Postcode......................Signed................................

HOW TO PAY

☐ I enclose a cheque/postal order for
£.......................... made payable to 'Tiptree Book Services'

☐ I wish to pay by Access/Visa/Switch/Delta card (delete where appropriate)

Card Number ☐☐☐☐☐☐☐☐☐☐☐☐☐☐☐☐
Expiry Date ☐☐☐☐

Post order to **TBS Direct, Tiptree Book Services, St. Lukes Chase, Tiptree, Essex, CO5 0SR.**

POSTAGE AND PACKING ARE FREE. Offer open in Great Britain including Northern Ireland. Books should arrive less than 28 days after we receive your order; they are subject to availability at time of ordering. If not entirely satisfied return in the same packaging and condition as received with a covering letter within 7 days. Vermilion books are available from all good booksellers.